Living and working with schizophrenia

Living and working with schizophrenia

Second edition

J.J. JEFFRIES

E. PLUMMER

M.V. SEEMAN

J.F. THORNTON

UNIVERSITY OF TORONTO PRESS
Toronto Buffalo London

First edition
© University of Toronto Press 1982
Reprinted 1983, 1984, 1985

Second edition
© University of Toronto Press 1990
Toronto Buffalo London
Printed in Canada

ISBN 0-8020-6781-6

Canadian Cataloguing in Publication Data

Main entry under title:
Living and working with schizophrenia

2nd ed.
Includes bibliographical references.
ISBN 0-8020-6781-6

1. Schizophrenia – Popular works. I. Jeffries, J. Joel, 1939–

RC514.J44 1990   616.89'82   C89-090744-7

To the memory of Sebastian K. Littmann, who devoted his life to working on behalf of the ill.

Contents

Foreword

I am schizophrenic, and I have been to asked to write a foreword to this book because my first book, *The Butterfly Ward*, a collection of short stories, dealt with schizophrenia.

I believe that I have been a schizophrenic since I was a child. Schizophrenics have lucid states, but when they are not lucid, life is sheer hell: raging all day and spending the night on a bed in a semi-catatonic state, hearing voices and seeing things that no one else can hear or see – the sharp edge of a razor ripping open flesh like a ripe grape, the smell of burning flesh. And all this is you but not you – at that moment illusion is all that exists; you have opened the door into another reality to which you alone hold the key. There are days, months, years when the world spins off its axis and no one can enter. We think we recognize someone we have known for years, we see the person's face in a dozen people only to realize (sometimes too late) that it is someone else.

I began to dream in another language at approximately the age of nine (although not all schizophrenics do this), and this language was not of Earth. When this language entered the world's arena and was found to be unacceptable, I ceased speaking for seven years. There are many beings that have crowded my other-worldly state. A painting of one hangs in my living room to remind me that if there is a nemesis then the world or half-world that I have chosen to live in is indeed it.

There are certain chairs one must not sit on, knocks on doors when there is no one there, eyes mysteriously blackened in the dark of day.

I have seen Satan, an angel disguised as a taxi driver, and run through the snow in stocking feet with my three-year-old son because it was not 1976 any longer. An hourglass was overturned (it was some time during the Second World War) and planes were strafing, ready to kill. The rest of my family, my parents, sisters, and brother, were crumpled and dried like old autumn leaves. Only my son and I were left alive searching for the underground where we would be safe with others who were not the enemy. There is a sensation of sitting in a chair talking to someone and feeling that you are separate and drifting, sitting in the chair beside yourself. Limbs become detached and floating and certain colors take on special meanings as do certain objects. I realize that all these are very personal experiences and that each schizophrenic has his own private key to other worlds.

My father once said sadly, wearily, 'She has been in so many institutions that we have lost count.' There are always those, the ones that we leave behind, family. Families that wait with dying hope and patience for months, years; families who give up waiting altogether. The son or daughter, mother or father, ceases to exist except perhaps as a piece of furniture stored away in some warehouse. One thing I would like to say to the families: while a schizophrenic is present, do not talk about him as if he does not exist. We are there, we are always there; we have ears just like everyone else.

There are good institutions and bad institutions, and the same can be said of psychiatrists. Despite Freud, who made great inroads into the cerebral ridges, and despite Jung and Adler and more recently Laing, psychiatry has a lot to learn. Psychiatry is Columbus in search of a key to the mind. Sometimes the key is found and a Pandora's box is opened, but then there is the further problem of dealing with the gargoyles that emerge. I was fortunate enough to have an excellent and caring psychiatrist for many years, despite the advice of one analyst who said to my family, 'Forget about her, she is hopelessly insane.' Today I am a 30-year-old single parent who owns her own house and takes care of a son, aged six. My family did not forget that I was alive and fighting and always there. Chemotherapy has been of great help to schizophrenics. I know that without my medication (and I was taken off it once by a behaviorist psychiatrist), I can neither eat nor sleep nor function in any way at all. Without drugs I am not of this world.

With the help of a good and caring psychiatrist I managed to make a life for myself and my six-year-old son. I have accepted my illness and used it in books, but I also do that with many experiences. I realize not every schizophrenic can write, but you can remain alive and fighting, for there are good psychiatrists and effective medications. You must take it on the jaw and pick yourself up again. I know that we are a bunch of punch-drunk fighters.

I am not 'cured,' but my condition is greatly improved. I live and function on the outside. This is not to say that living on the outside of an institution is 'fun' or 'easy.' It is not. If you are a schizophrenic, you will find that the loneliness can be appalling, like living in solitary confinement. You may work with others and find that they do not talk to you, perhaps because your speech is disjointed or you are actually shy. You may live in a neighborhood for years without acquiring a single friend. It may seem that you live and move among people as one who is invisible. It will not be easy to go back to your family, for they may regard you as a stranger, as in fact you are to them. It will take them a long time to regard you as something less than an enigma. They may always regard you as an enigma. But it is all worth it. You can find pleasure in things that other people take for granted. I still take pleasure in shopping for groceries, in sitting in restaurants, in going to movies. And when you find a friend, and you will, cherish that friend, for he is better than gold. And you are as alive and valuable as anyone else in this world. It is nice to know that what you are feeling you are *really* feeling.

There is also something good and shining about this disease. It gives us a rare insight into the world that few people have. There are people who know we are alive and care. Try to let the world know that we matter. We matter a hell of a lot.

MARGARET GIBSON

Preface

Schizophrenia is a serious mental illness. The odds that a person will develop this illness at some time in life are one in a hundred. It strikes most frequently in late adolescence or early adulthood, a time of great expectations in our lives, and it can shatter those expectations by running a prolonged and rocky course. Not only victims but also families and friends are affected by schizophrenia, each in different ways. Their sufferings are immeasurable, as are the social and financial costs to communities at large.

The illness was first described a long time ago and we know that it occurs throughout the world. We do not yet, however, understand precisely the cause or causes of schizophrenia, although research is progressing rapidly. In the early years of studying schizophrenia, researchers explored all possibilities – physical factors, genetic inheritance, biochemical aberrations, social factors, and psychological explanations. Investigation today still ranges just as widely. Since the schizophrenic's distress is often accompanied by disruption in the lives of the members of his family, some researchers assumed that the family disruption came first. They maintained that schizophrenic symptoms arose as an attempt to ward off the disrupting influence of family members. This led to the false conclusion that the family played a causative role in the illness – a heavy burden for a family to bear.

Even without this, the condition imposes an extraordinary burden on the person afflicted and on the family he belongs to. Since the family, by and large, continues to assume the largest management and support role in the individual's prolonged struggle against schizophrenia, it became time for the health and social service professions to stop alienating families by drawing false conclusions about the cause of schizophrenia and, instead, to increase and bolster family resources. At long last, professional efforts are now being made to organize support systems for families of schizophrenics.

The authors, who have all been actively involved in the care and study of schizophrenic patients both in hospitals and in private offices, began to address this problem through the establishment of relatives' groups. Recalling similar work done with families of tuberculosis patients earlier this century, we assumed that groups could play an educational, a supportive, and a motivational role for the relatives and friends of schizophrenics. It became clear to us in the groups that many relatives (and patients) had little accurate information about schizophrenia: about its origin, manifestations, course, treatment, outcome, and risks.

In the past, health professionals, faced with their own uncertain knowledge about all these aspects of schizophrenia, were understandably reluctant to speak freely and openly to patients and relatives about the illness. They felt, for the most part, that 'the less you mention, the less it hurts.'

This approach, we feel, needs to be modified, and our efforts at organizing groups of relatives, holding public meetings, and writing this book – all with the express aim of talking more openly about schizophrenia – are attempts to restructure attitudes towards this illness.

This book is composed of many questions and answers – all of which arose in our clinical work with patients and relatives. Also included, in Part Two, are autobiographical accounts of problems and solutions.

We have chosen, quite arbitrarily, to refer to the patient as 'he,' although, it must be made clear, women are as prone to the illness as men.

We hope that this book will be of most help to those who already have firsthand knowledge of what it is like to live with schizophrenia but who feel a need to know more. It is not a textbook, but a practical reference book for those whom professionals sometimes refer to as 'lay people.' In real life, it is those very lay people who can and do, on a daily basis, contribute to smoothing the path towards a happier life for the schizophrenic patient. Professionals, in contrast, monitor and advise from the more remote locations of their hospitals, clinics, and private offices.

We express our deep appreciation to the patients and relatives who contributed to this book. We are particularly grateful to those who asked questions, and demanded answers.

Acknowledgments

There have been many advertent and inadvertent contributors to this book. Special thanks go to Ms Margaret James, Ms Bernadette Monsegue, the Clarke Institute Parents and Friends of Schizophrenia, Mrs Claire McLaughlin, and Ontario Friends of Schizophrenics.

PART ONE
Basic Information

ONE

What is schizophrenia?

How was schizophrenia discovered?

The name *schizophrenia* was introduced in 1911 by a Swiss psychiatrist, Eugen Bleuler. In 1896 a German psychiatrist, Emil Kraepelin, had named the illness *dementia praecox* (early brain loss), thinking it led to a deterioration of the personality at a fairly early age. Bleuler disagreed. He observed that a loss of mental functioning did not invariably develop. The new name, *schizophrenia*, comes from the Greek *skhizo*, to split, and *phren*, mind. Bleuler wanted to emphasize a basic split or loss of connectedness in the personality. This split could take the form of a faulty association of ideas, an inappropriate expression of emotion, a detachment from reality, or all of these. It is now apparent that schizophrenia has a variety of forms for each of which there are somewhat different symptoms and for which there may even be different causes.

Who can become schizophrenic?

Everyone, in any part of the world, has a 1 percent chance of developing schizophrenia some time in his life. The manifestations of the illness, however, are to some extent influenced by the culture a person lives in. Thus the false belief (delusion) that one is Jesus is much more likely to be held by someone in a Christian culture; the impression of being controlled by external electrical impulses occurs more readily in people who live in countries where there is electricity. The illness occurs in both sexes and makes its first appearance most commonly when an individual is in his twenties. There are rarer forms that appear in early childhood or in later life. The illness occurs in all walks of life, but once affected, people tend to drift downwards socially and often end up living in the poorer sections of their communities. In part this is a result of moving away from home to be independent, and suffering the consequences of unemployment, recurrent hospitalization, and loss of vocational skills. Poverty and hardship are associated with the illness but seem to be results, not causes.

What is an illness?

An illness shows itself through symptoms and signs. Symptoms are unpleasant, painful, or unusual experiences; rarely, they are pleasurable and produce an unrealistic sense of well-being. Signs, in contrast, are changes in behavior or demeanor that can be noticed by others. Both symptoms and signs may be physical or mental or both. They may occur suddenly and may be severe; they are then called *acute*. Or they may develop insidiously, sometimes over a number of years. When they remain for a long period of time they are called *chronic*. A chronic condition happens most often after the individual has experienced several acute episodes.

Another way of looking at the symptoms and signs of schizophrenia is to label them *positive* or *negative*. For example, the hearing of voices when there is no one speaking in the vicinity (hallucination of hearing) or severe agitation is a positive change: though unwelcome, they are *additions* to the person's usual behavior. Negative symptoms are *losses*, such as the lessened drive to get things done or the diminished ability to derive pleasure from social activities. Studies have shown that the positive symptoms are more likely than the others to ease with medical treatment.

What are the main features of a schizophrenic illness?

To diagnose schizophrenia is not always an easy task because the features show up gradually and are not dramatic. The diagnosis can be made with confidence only when the patient is fully co-operative and not intoxicated or when the symptoms are quite advanced. Symptoms may include:

Delusions: A person may have an absolutely certain conviction (*delusion*) that: a) his thoughts are being influenced, controlled, inserted into his head, or broadcast; b) events around him have particular significance for him; c) he is being persecuted or treated unfairly, discriminated against, or subject to special treatment; d) he has special powers or importance; and/or e) his body is changed or is being moved or influenced by an outside agency.

Thought disorder: The logical process of thought is lost.

Auditory hallucinations: A person may experience: a) his thoughts being spoken aloud; b) a voice talking about him, commenting on his behavior; and/or c) a voice or voices talking to him.

Disturbances of feeling: A person may exhibit a) incongruous or inappropriate feeling, e.g., laughing for no apparent reason or when talking about sad events; b) flatness of affect, meaning that his range of emotion is limited; and/or c) loss of ability to make or maintain personal relationships.

Physical symptoms: These can include: a) a slowness of movements, withdrawal, and reclusiveness; b) severe overactivity; c) adoption of strange postures and manneristic behavior. (The last two have, for unknown reasons, become increasing rare over the last 30 years.)

A distinct break in the patient's life: This can take the form of a definite behavioral or personality change.

A diagnosis of schizophrenia is not readily made when there is marked sadness and depression or when there is evidence of recent drug use, especially of LSD or other hallucinogens, cocaine, amphetamines, hashish, or marijuana. It must, of course, be realized that such drugs are sometimes used by the schizophrenic to alleviate subjective distress. They may, at times, help to bring on the illness in a vulnerable individual.

The diagnosis is often easier when the onset of changes in behavior is acute. Unfortunately there is also some evidence that the person who becomes ill more slowly and insidiously is also the one who responds less well to the various methods of treatment used today. Accurate diagnosis requires professional training and experience.

What are the causes of schizophrenia?

Much has been written about the probable causes of schizophrenia. Many theories have had to be discarded because they were arrived at too quickly, without proper scientific inquiry. For example, in Victorian times some seriously blamed masturbation for the development of all kinds of insanity including schizophrenia. Later theories blamed improper nutrition and advocated large doses of vitamins. Other researchers thought they found a cause in faulty communication within families; later it became clear that problems in communication (e.g. the 'double bind' – a message from one person to another containing contradictory expectations) could be found in practically all families. The discovery of a so-called *pink spot* on the chromatographs obtained from the urine of schizophrenic patients created great hopes of a chemical breakthrough. It later became clear that the pink spot was related to the hospital diet of the patients tested. Current research is focused on identifying specific genes associated with the illness. A gene in chromosome 5 is being investigated.

Researchers follow many alleys: some lead forward; most do not. However, a few theories are generally accepted: for example, that a predisposition or vulnerability to schizophrenia may be passed from one generation to another (see page 11). Since the symptoms usually first appear in the second or even third decade and not at birth, an age-specific hormonal or developmental trigger is probably required for schizophrenia to occur.

Can stress cause schizophrenia?

There is little doubt that stress frequently contributes to the initial appearance or subsequent recurrence of illness. For example, careful studies have shown that a schizophrenic relapse frequently occurs in someone who is threatened with the loss of his job. Such a relapse is also more likely when the person lives in a highly charged emotional environment where he is frequently exposed to critical evaluation from those around him. Such stress produces recurrence of stomach ulcers in one person, skin rashes in another, alcoholism in a third, and schizophrenia in yet others. A possible way of understanding schizophrenia is to consider that stress produces biochemical changes in the body that the brain cells cannot deal with adequately. Current research focuses on a trans-mitter substance in the brain known as dopamine. Some research-ers suspect that certain brain cells in the schizophrenic may be oversensitive to dopamine; others suspect that some of the neces-sary mechanisms to neutralize dopamine are lacking. Currently it seems that schizophrenia has a definite inherited basis, but that its onset may be triggered by stress.

The outlook is not nearly as grim as some authors have sug-gested. It is important for the patient and his family to learn about the illness, for they can then cope more effectively. All those involved – patient, family, friends, therapist – should be clear about what the illness is and what it is not, and about what it implies about the past, the present, and the future. When patients, families, friends, and therapists work together the outlook becomes more favorable.

To tell or not to tell?

Many doctors, themselves uncertain, do not tell patients and family members that the diagnosis may be schizophrenia. The schizophrenic may, for example, exhibit signs that are indistinguishable from those related to certain drug-induced states experienced with LSD or amphetamine psychosis. Or the schizophrenic-like behavior may be an isolated reaction which, once over, never recurs. Until a firm diagnosis is reached, many doctors prefer not to talk openly about schizophrenia in order to save patients and families needless worry and concern. Yet experience has shown us that patients and families worry when they do not know. They are entitled to know at least the diagnostic possibilities, to be fully and expertly informed of the best preventive and treatment measures available, and to gain a hopeful and realistic view of the future, both immediate and long-term.

Even when the diagnosis is certain, many clinicians are hesitant to share this information with the patient and his family. They maintain that this particular diagnosis is still so ill-understood that informing the family of a schizophrenic may be harmful. It may provoke completely wrong conclusions. In the same way, some doctors are reluctant to use the word *cancer* even for the more treatable types of cancer because the word itself has such ominous connotations that the individuals involved become needlessly frightened. It is, of course, essential when giving the diagnosis to explain the illness and to stress the range of severity with which schizophrenia may strike. While it may make a person very ill indeed, in many instances the symptoms may be mild. It must also be explained that present-day treatments, while not cures, alleviate most of the symptoms and allow a qualitatively satisfying life. A full explanation is usually better than attempts at concealment.

Some diseases have developed a 'shameful' connotation, as if they were the results of poor hygiene or of sinful acts, something to be hidden from public view. Leprosy used to have this connotation before the world realized, through the work of Albert Schweitzer in Africa and Mother Teresa in India, that lepers are human beings and that the disease is relatively noncontagious, eminently curable, and definitely not the result of sin. Some infestations and sexually transmitted diseases, particularly AIDS, share this connotation of shame, as do certain mental disorders. While doctors themselves should not find any disease shameful, they are often sensitive to the public's view and make up the names for some diseases to protect the patient from needless humiliation. It is for this reason that individuals with schizophrenia may be told that they have suffered a 'nervous breakdown,' are 'under stress,' are 'suffering from exhaustion,' are 'going through an identity crisis,' or have a 'functional psychosis' or a 'reactive psychosis.' There are many other words and phrases that are used to protect the patient from a diagnostic label that is thought to be shameful. Our work has taught us that there is nothing shameful about schizophrenia. We would like the patient and his family to become familiar with it.

Some individuals refuse to use the diagnosis of schizophrenia because in some parts of the world political dissidents have been sent to mental hospitals, their 'illness' labeled officially as schizophrenia. In most parts of the world, however, the medical profession realizes that the illness, even though it affects the mind and the whole personality, is in many respects a diagnosis like pneumonia, rheumatic fever, or some other medical disorder. An ethical doctor would not use it to wield power or to repress unwelcome opinions. While it has in some quarters developed connotations of hopelessness, intractability, or shame, such a response is, for the most part, quite unjustified by modern experience.

When we refer in this book to schizophrenia or to schizophrenic we speak in the same way as we might when talking about diabetes and diabetic. In the same way that the statement 'He is diabetic' describes only that aspect of the person that has to do with a specific disease and his reactions to it, so 'He is schizophrenic' refers only to an individual's specific illness and his reactions to it. It says nothing about his personality, his intelligence, his morals, his interests, or any of the countless other qualities that make this person unique. It refers to an illness that, however unfortunate, can frequently be controlled and that may in the future be overcome.

Schizophrenia and childbearing

Across the world, in every culture and in every race, the probability of developing schizophrenia seems remarkably similar. That probability has long been considered to be about 1 in 100 for every child born, though some recent figures suggest that the rate may be even higher than this. Perhaps as much as 1.6 percent of the world's population is affected or one child in every 60. Sometimes schizophrenia will occur quite unexpectedly in somebody who has no family history of the illness at all. When there is a history of this illness in the family, however, the possibility of illness rises for close relatives. The amount by which it rises is unknown. We do know that about 4 percent of the general population is vulnerable to major depressive illness and another 1 percent to bipolar affective disorder (manic-depressive illness). We have to bear this in mind when we try to understand the meaning of the usually quoted statistic that the child of a schizophrenic has a 1 in 10 chance of becoming psychotic in adult life. A little over half the cases of psychosis in the children of schizophrenics turn out to be schizophrenia. The other half turn out to be mood disorders and this appears to be about the same as in the rest of the population. Thus, while there *is* an increased occurrence of schizophrenia in first-degree relatives, it seems that this represents only a fivefold increase over what one would normally expect if the illness occurred randomly. Just as parents and their children share 50 percent of their genes, so do siblings, and thus the chance of schizophrenia in the sibling of a schizophrenic, once said to be 10 percent, is again inflated by the misidentification of people who, in fact, have a mood disorder.

It is important to realize that this extra risk for close relatives has nothing to do with living together. Children born to a schizophrenic parent, but adopted out at birth, have exactly the same risk of developing schizophrenia as those raised by their schizophrenic parent. Similarly, children who are adopted by a parent who develops schizophrenia do not suffer an increased risk of schizophrenia, even if they grow up with the schizophrenic adoptive parent. This seems to make it clear that the illness is fundamentally biological, and although the mode of inheritance is not known, it certainly seems that a vulnerability is being inherited. Against this we must balance the knowledge that merely having a genetic propensity for this illness is not sufficient. For example, even if a person has schizophrenia, the risk for an identical twin is only 40 percent. This seems to be true even when the twins are brought up in a very similar environment, as most identical twins are. It has been possible to trace some rare cases of identical twins brought up separately and, in these instances, should one twin develop schizophrenia, the rate in the other one stays at 40 percent. If twins are fraternal (nonidentical) and one has schizophrenia, the other has the same chance of becoming ill as any other brother or sister, that is, less than 10 percent.

The risk seems to be very low once we move a further generation away. For many years the likelihood of developing the disease for a grandchild, aunt, uncle, nephew, or niece of a schizophrenic was given as about 3 percent. It may be even less than this. Indeed it seems to be little more than the occurrence in the general population. An individual with schizophrenia in the family has to bear in mind that age is important in determining vulnerability. Men are most likely to develop schizophrenia from age 15 to 25, whereas for women it tends to occur between age 20 and 30. After the age of 35, the chance of schizophrenia occurring for the first time is very small indeed.

In marriages where one of the parents is schizophrenic, the genetic risk to the unborn child must be considered before embarking on parenthood. Also important is the potential hardship for the parents-to-be. During pregnancy it is common for mothers to worry about the future prospects for their child, and it is especially stressful to be concerned about bearing a child who is at risk for a serious illness.

Although the neuroleptic drugs have not been shown to cause serious damage to the fetus, in principle one should take no drugs at all when pregnant. Even drugs that have had a good safety record should be avoided because of potential long-term effects on the unborn child. Therefore, if one is or is planning to become pregnant, antipsychotic medication should probably be stopped if the risks associated with relapse are not excessive. This does put the mother at some risk for a flare-up of the illness, though some women have found that their illness goes into remission during pregnancy. Childbirth is a particularly stressful experience, because it is accompanied by major hormonal changes. This may contribute to the triggering of a schizophrenic episode in the mother. Perhaps most important of all is the demand that the infant places on the parents. The demands of a young child are continuous and this kind of nonstop responsibility may be very hard for somebody who has a degree of disability from schizophrenia. Unless there are substantial family and financial supports, being a parent can be an exceptionally difficult task for individuals who suffer from schizophrenia.

Adopted children

Nowadays it has been increasingly common for single women who have become pregnant to keep their child and, with the aid of social agencies, to raise the child alone. This has led, in some parts of the world, to a real shortage of children available for adoption; so much so that many people have gone to third world countries in order to adopt children. When a child does become available for adoption in our affluent society, it indicates that some problem exists for the parents. In some cities in the United States, children are commonly given up for adoption because their mothers are addicted to drugs. Another reason to give up a child for adoption may be mental illness, and it is therefore increasingly common for prospective adoptive parents to want to know about schizophrenia. A couple from Toronto adopted two girls. One of the girls developed a schizo-affective disorder and the other developed schizo-phrenia. One would think that the chance of this happening randomly would be about 1 in 10,000, but probably the risk is greater than this because of the increased likelihood that children offered for adoption have a maternal history of schizophrenia.

When prospective parents do have the opportunity to adopt the child of a schizophrenic mother, they have to take the risk to the child into account. Good parenting may reduce but will not reverse that risk so that prospective parents may be committing themselves to a child who later will develop a serious mental illness despite any precaution they take. Many parents adopt children who are already handicapped. This is perhaps easier, however, than raising children who are healthy and happy and who subsequently develop schizophrenia. In any event, a serious illness such as this is made easier to bear in the context of a supportive, committed family.

TWO

Inpatient treatment

Is hospitalization always necessary?

Hospitals are not as a rule considered happy places. Most people do not like the idea of leaving their home and entering the hospital. No matter what the illness, hospitalization is an exceptional step.

Why then admit a schizophrenic to the hospital? A doctor may recommend admission to hospital because the patient has an acute and severe illness that requires intensive observation and care. Or the patient may exhibit signs and symptoms that the doctor cannot readily explain or that constitute a possible risk to safety and health. Even when the person is not acutely ill, the doctor may arrange an elective admission in order to observe and study the illness. The general advantages of hospitalization are: expert observation and care for an acutely ill patient and investigation of less acute symptoms in a planned and systematic manner. In psychiatry, the hospital is also used to 'cool' things, for example, when a serious quarrel has disrupted family life. At other times, patients are admitted to hospital simply because they are homeless and in need of shelter. Criteria for hospital admission differ somewhat from community to community, and from hospital to hospital.

All these considerations are involved in deciding whether or not a schizophrenic patient should be admitted to hospital. Outpatient assessment and treatment are possible provided that the condition is not too severe, the doctor has a good appreciation of the situation, and the doctor and patient know each other well. However, a person experiencing the first attack of acute schizophrenia is apt to be very disorganized and frightened; his behavior can be quite erratic and upsetting. Predictions of dangerousness to self and others are difficult to make. Inpatient treatment in such conditions is desirable. But to be admitted, a person must agree to enter the hospital. If he disagrees, the doctor will have to decide whether, without hospital care, there is risk of the person physically harming himself or others seriously.

Legal requirements must be met before a person can be hospitalized against his will. The necessary conditions vary from country to country, province to province, and state to state. By and large, the criteria have become increasingly strict over recent years. In most communities, there must be evidence of mental illness and the risk of physical harm before an unwilling person can be admitted. Involuntary admissions are made only on the recommendation of a physician, who will rely on his examination of the patient and on the details furnished by the family. Admission, however, is not the same as treatment. Admitted patients may still refuse treatment. In countries with modern mental health legislation, *treatment* against a person's will requires approval of an appeal board, although in emergencies a designated proxy may be asked for permission to administer a given treatment (see page 82).

The hospital staff

Wards vary in size. There are single- and multi-bed rooms, and some hospitals may still have dormitories. The ward is usually built around the nursing station, which is in the charge of the head nurse. Each ward also has a sitting room and eating facilities, as well as group and recreation rooms and shower and washroom facilities. Psychiatric wards, by and large, are not very private places.

The staff belong to various health disciplines. They include registered nurses and nursing assistants, clinical psychologists and social workers, occupational and recreational therapists. They usually work under the overall direction of a qualified psychiatrist. Teamwork has become the norm, with each team responsible for a small number of patients, and with each patient assigned for his main therapy to one or more team members. In teaching hospitals psychiatric residents will be much in evidence. They are qualified medical doctors who are undergoing specialty training in psychiatry. Students of the various disciplines (medicine, nursing, social work, occupational therapy, psychology, pharmacy, and divinity) also spend some of their time attached to a psychiatric ward. There is also the support staff, including secretaries, receptionists, kitchen personnel, cleaners, and, in some instances, security personnel. Most staff offices are located on or near a ward, but this varies from hospital to hospital.

The routine of a ward is a reflection of the team orientation and of the philosophy of the hospital. One of the basic routines deals with the necessity of creating an environment which, although artificial and restrictive, is nevertheless health-promoting. In addition there is the need for observation of patients who may at times be very ill and at risk. There is often a system of ward privileges. This system defines the degree of freedom of the individual patient on the ward. The very ill patient may be restricted to his room with a staff member present on a round-the-clock basis. At the other extreme is the patient who may come and go as he pleases as long as he informs the staff of his plans.

When a patient enters such a ward system, it is important for him and his family to be given information about the ward routine. When this is not done early on, unwelcome surprises are sometimes in store for patient, family, and staff alike.

The initial examination

On admission to the ward, the patient can expect both a physical as well as a psychiatric examination by a doctor. The psychiatric examination may last an hour or more and is intended to allow the doctor or therapist to get a comprehensive view of the person's circumstances and, in particular, of recent changes. It will include questions about the onset and development of the illness, family relationships, school and work, previous health record and treatments received before. Most important, an attempt is made by the doctor to understand how the patient's mind and feelings are working at that particular time. This is done partly by observation and simple questions and partly by a number of more searching questions, some of them quite personal. Psychological tests may later be administered by clinical psychologists to help the clinician in his diagnosis and in the planning of appropriate treatment.

The physical examination is a general check of all bodily systems, but specialized examinations may be recommended when appropriate and these are then performed by other consulting specialists. Blood and urine are tested routinely. Additional tests such as X-rays, electrocardiograms, and electroencephalograms (brain-wave recordings) may also be carried out. They are indicated when symptoms overlap with those of other medical conditions.

Relatives or friends who accompany the patient to the hospital may be interviewed. The information they give is used in trying to understand the illness and the patient's social relationships.

Some hospitals have a special admission ward; after an initial period there, the patient may be transferred to a longer-stay ward.

The diagnosis

Usually schizophrenia is fairly easy to diagnose by the time somebody is hospitalized. In fact the diagnosis may already have been made. On occasion there is uncertainty, and the patient may need a period of observation. There is no specific test for schizophrenia and there may be times when the doctor is not absolutely sure of the diagnosis. The patient and family need to trust the doctor's judgment, so, if they have doubts they should ask for a second opinion. A good doctor will always be willing to have another doctor provide a consultation.

Some doctors, however, are not at ease when it comes to sharing a diagnosis of schizophrenia with their patients, believing that the information may upset them. In our experience it is probably more upsetting to be kept in the dark for any length of time or to be left imagining that the doctor does not know what is wrong. Sometimes the doctor is willing to share the diagnosis, but the patient is not willing to accept it. It is, after all, not easy to accept that one is 'mentally ill.' It is very important for the patient to know that schizophrenia is an illness, that it is treatable, and that his co-operation will hasten the recovery process.

Diagnostic alternatives

Schizophrenia is not the easiest diagnosis to pin down. As a patient it is very frustrating to be treated as if one were schizophrenic without the diagnosis being definite. This happens because the differentiation of schizophrenia from other major mental disorders is not always clear. There are no specific diagnostic tests. There is only the clinical judgment of the psychiatrist, and for that reason it is often wise to get a second opinion from a skilled specialist.

What are the alternatives? Certainly the most likely source of confusion is that the person does not have schizophrenia but in fact has a bipolar affective disorder. This is the condition which was formerly called manic-depression. Particularly in adolescence, the presentation of the acute psychotic episode may be very similar in these two diseases. The possibility that this is a mood disorder rather than schizophrenia increases with the following symptoms: elation, severe depression, frequent mood swings, wearing bright clothing, frequent changes of clothing, increased interest in sex, increased spending, great energy with minimal need for sleep. Often the distinction between these two illnesses cannot be made until some years have passed and a pattern develops. The situation is complicated by the fact that the neuroleptic drugs, which treat schizophrenia, may also effectively treat mania; so even if the diagnosis is wrong, the person may respond well. It is ultimately important to make this diagnostic distinction because the course of the two disorders differs, and mood disorders may be prevented by specific treatment.

Another source of confusion is what is nowadays called delusional disorder. This is an illness very similar to schizophrenia in which the predominant symptoms are delusional ideas. Usually thought disorder is absent or minimal, and auditory hallucinations are infrequent. This illness often occurs later in life than schizophrenia. It tends to 'breed true' so that other family members will have suffered from delusional disorders as well. The neuroleptic drugs are effective in delusional disorder. In fact, treatment of the two conditions is very similar.

A very difficult diagnostic distinction to make is that between a drug-induced psychosis and schizophrenia. This is particularly true in a young population which has a heavy use of drugs. Psychoses can be triggered by amphetamines, cocaine, LSD and other hallucinogens, hashish, and marijuana. Any of these drugs can cause an illness that mimics schizophrenia. What makes it all the more difficult is that the people who are developing schizophrenia may also be abusing drugs. Thus we may be seeing a drug-induced psychosis that looks like schizophrenia or a schizophrenic illness that has been made worse by the use of drugs and there is no sure way of knowing the difference. Recent research has suggested that heavy users of marijuana have an increased risk of schizophrenia. It is possible that young people developing schizophrenia have a tendency to use marijuana more, but that is less likely than the alternative theory, which is that the excessive indulgence in marijuana increases the likelihood of schizophrenia in those genetically predisposed.

The question of brain disease is often raised. In fact, confusion between schizophrenia and brain tumors or other disorders of the brain is very rare indeed. One illness that can mimic schizophrenia is temporal lobe epilepsy, otherwise known as psychomotor epilepsy, but in practice it is rarely a significant alternative. An even more remote possibility is a very rare form of the metabolic disease porphyria.

The choice of treatment

Usually the admitting doctor decides on a provisional plan of management and treatment. It may include any or all of: medication, activity programs, behavioral programs, group and individual discussions, exploratory individual and family therapy, and general supervision. Within a few days of admission there is a meeting of staff members involved in the patient's care, and a comprehensive plan of treatment is drawn up. One of the staff will then meet with the patient to discuss this plan and its implications and to seek his reactions and co-operation. Not infrequently the patient himself has good ideas about what will be of help to him and he should feel free to draw the staff's attention to these ideas.

Medication

Chapter 4 and Appendix III describe the role of drug therapy in schizophrenia and give detailed information about the various types of medication currently in use, as well as about dosages.

ECT

Electroconvulsive treatment (electroshock therapy) has had some bad press in recent years, particularly under the impact of movies like *One Flew over the Cuckoo's Nest*. It is, however, a safe and humane treatment that has been found to be particularly effective for people with severe depressions. It may also help some schizophrenics, especially those who respond poorly to drugs and who, as the result of their disordered thinking and feelings, are severely disorganized, cannot eat, or are suicidal. Physical complications are very rare since great care is taken to ensure a thorough physical examination of the patient prior to treatment and good general anesthesia, including a muscle relaxant. Patients used to experience memory loss during the course of the treatment; the memory usually returned to normal within about two weeks. Modern ECT machines use less current and cause only mild and transitory memory disturbances. Some experts claim that medications make ECT unnecessary in schizophrenia but there continue to be many occasions when ECT is life-saving. When needed, it is a valuable treatment.

Miscellaneous physical treatments

Many treatments have been used for schizophrenia. These have included hot baths and cold baths, wet packs and dry packs (a pack is a sheet wrapped around the individual to keep him immobile), vitamins, insulin coma, starvation, dialysis, and a vast variety of drugs and diets. Most of these have been discarded. New treatment ideas always arise and they must be investigated because one of them may turn out to be a breakthrough. However, patients and families should be wary of novel, untested treatments because they may delay the beginning of effective therapy. If experimental treatments are offered, the patient should ask for a second opinion.

Psychological treatments

Understanding and acceptance of the condition and reassurance from others are important ingredients of hospital care. Initially, unnecessary stimulation is avoided. Gradually, more responsibility and decision-making is introduced. In some instances, psychosocial and behavioral programs help the patient to reintegrate into society by systematically rewarding socially appropriate behavior.

As the patient recovers, he may benefit from a form of psychotherapy which allows expression of feelings about what has happened to him. It will help him to come to terms with the sense of shock and loss that is associated with having gone through a psychotic illness. To have such an illness is a major blow to self-esteem and some people may deal with it by pretending that it never happened. It is best to be able to talk about it openly, to express how distressing it is, and to grieve the perceived loss of sanity. The patient can then move from there to constructive planning for the future.

Family therapy

The family continues to be important in the treatment of schizophrenia. Family therapy was particularly popular years ago, when some psychiatrists thought that schizophrenia was caused by family problems. This is no longer considered to be a reasonable theory. However, nowadays family education about the illness is a very important component in management, as is counseling about how best to interact with the patient, particularly upon the patient's return home from hospital. This counseling may need to be over an extended period. More rarely there may be need for ongoing family therapy. This will occur in those circumstances where stresses within the family magnify the distress caused by the illness to provide a situation that perpetuates the patient's disability or causes family dysfunction. Such therapy will not deal directly with the schizophrenic illness, but will help family members to cope more effectively.

Financial affairs

As a rule, hospitalized psychiatric patients are able to maintain control of their finances, although hospital regulations usually demand that valuables or large sums of money be deposited in the hospital business office for safekeeping. When the psychiatric disorder is of such a degree and nature that irreparable financial harm may result, the psychiatrist has the power to declare the person financially incompetent. The patient's assets are then managed by a private committee (often a relative) or by the public trustee (see page 72).

Visiting regulations

Psychiatric wards welcome visitors and usually have generous visiting hours. Restrictions apply at certain times so as to avoid interference with ward programs such as therapy, meals, and sleep. However, visiting hours and rules depend upon the philosophy of the ward and its patient population, with a good deal of variation from ward to ward. On some occasions visiting may be seriously disturbing to the patient or to the visitor, and the staff may temporarily suspend visits or limit their duration.

Family contact with staff

Each psychiatric facility tends to have its own unique communication system and it is important for those visiting a relative or friend to find out about the organization of the unit. Sometimes the family is expected to contact the doctor, sometimes the social worker, and sometimes the nurse. Some units are flexible, and all the staff can be approached. It is, however, very important to find out the norms for each particular place. There should be at least one person whom you can contact on a regular basis to get updates on the progress of the patient. This may be somebody you can speak to whenever you come for a visit, or you may need to arrange for a special interview in person or by telephone.

On occasion you may hear complaints about treatment from the patient. It is important to discuss these complaints with the staff. They may be a product of the patient's misinterpretations or a failing on the part of the staff that must be remedied. Most often they are a result of misunderstanding between patient and staff. If the family or a friend is concerned that the treatment is inadequate, they should ask for a second opinion, preferably from a psychiatrist outside the hospital. Alternatively, they may ask for a transfer to another facility. This may not, however, always be feasible. The other facility may not be willing to take patients on transfer and it may therefore be necessary to work out any difficulties in communication or understanding with the staff of the unit where the patient is hospitalized.

Passes

A patient whose illness is not too severe is given the opportunity to leave the hospital to spend a weekend with family or friends, to go out to dinner or a show, or to attend significant family functions. The success of these outings reflects the extent to which recovery has progressed. Whether a patient is ready to resume the activities of everyday life can be judged by how well the visits go. After an outing, it is important for the patient to report back his observations about how well he managed. If anything significant did occur, it is often helpful for the family or friends to let the staff know.

As a general rule, a pass should be seen as part of a gradual convalescence and not as an intense social engagement. Whenever necessary, guidance should be sought from the ward staff as to what is advisable. It is safer for a patient on medication not to drive, drink, or go near machinery when on a pass unless specifically given permission to do so by the treating physician.

Of course, not every pass goes smoothly, and if the patient feels upset or if his behavior is disturbing to those with whom he is spending his time, it is perfectly appropriate to return to the hospital early rather than to let things get out of control.

Other illnesses

All psychiatric units have arrangements available for medical and surgical consultation at short notice, and the patient is usually assured of competent medical help for any other illness that occurs while in hospital.

Discharge planning

A short hospital stay is generally to be preferred, because people who are hospitalized for a long time have great difficulty in returning to their previous level of activity. This is true whatever the illness. Too often passivity is induced by hospitalization and can make being an 'invalid' attractive and resuming the full activities of life unappealing. However, some patients respond rather slowly to treatment. The psychiatric staff has very difficult decisions to make in balancing adequate control of the symptoms and speedy discharge.

The final decision about discharge is based on a number of factors. These include the degree to which the symptoms have disappeared, the patient's social functioning on his weekend passes, and the extent to which an adequate follow-up has been organized. The length of stay varies a great deal. The average for a first schizophrenic illness is about six weeks.

It is also very important for the staff to consider the emotional environment to which the patient will return. Recent research has shown that patients who return to homes where there is a high degree of emotional expression, particularly of a critical nature, break down and return to the hospital more readily. However, this is true only when the patient is spending a lot of time at home in close contact with family members. Too much closeness may be a cause of tension and upset for all the family (and not just in schizophrenia). It is not a cause of schizophrenia, but it can lead to stress and breakdown and readmission to hospital.

There are various ways to deal with discharge from hospital. The patient may decide not to return to the family home and arrangements can be made for a new living situation. Whether or not the patient returns home he will probably fare better if he is occupied outside the house most weekdays, for example, in a day hospital, workshop, school, or job. Also, in those families where there is a lot of emotion and criticism, family counseling will often help to reduce the family tension and ease the situation for all the family members.

A comprehensive discharge plan should cover medication, therapy, job planning, living arrangements, financial planning, and social activity. The plan should be drawn up by the hospital team, the patient, his family, and the post-hospital community team. Families can be crucial here in examining and deciding on possible options.

Day care or evening care?

Many psychiatric wards have day care programs. These are intended mainly for patients ready to be discharged from inpatient care who may require a period of less intense involvement. Day patients usually attend on weekdays during working hours. In some settings they simply follow the general ward timetable. In others a special program has been developed for day patients with perhaps a focus on their particular problems.

A different type of day care is offered in certain specialized settings where admission to an intensive five- or seven-day-a-week day (only) care program is seen as an alternative to inpatient care. There is much to be said for such programs for they allow people to remain in their familiar surroundings and thus avoid the stigma that results from patients no longer being visible among their peers or friends.

Evening care is another variety of partial hospitalization. It is particularly appropriate for patients who are ready to return to work or to school, but who are concerned about their ability to adjust, especially during the first week or two after discharge from the ward. For these patients, evening or night care permits a solution. The patient is away from the ward all day, either at work or at school, and returns to the ward for the evening meal. It is desirable that special treatment programs be arranged for such patients at hours convenient to them.

Patient advocates

It is increasingly common for governments to place patient advocates in psychiatric hospitals. The psychiatric patient is seen as requiring special protection and civil libertarians are particularly concerned about the rights of psychotic patients, most of whom are schizophrenic. There are some who consider that psychiatrists abuse the power vested in them to control patients when necessary and that psychiatrists are therefore at times abrogating patients' rights. It is the patient advocate's task to inform the patient of his civil rights. The patient might have a right to refuse medication or to appeal commitment and it is of course important that the patient be aware of this. Ideally, the patient advocate is helpful and useful. There are, however, occasional stories heard of advocates who view the psychiatrist as an oppressor and urge the patient to resist him in any way possible. The patient may then effectively sabotage any attempts at therapy. This may turn out to be a disaster for the patient who remains psychotic and hospitalized, deprived of the opportunity for treatment. There are other settings in which the advocate and the psychiatrist have achieved an appropriate collaboration despite opposing viewpoints. If the patient or the family feel that the psychiatrist or some other member of the psychiatric staff is abusing power, the advocate will advise them on how to proceed. If, as sometimes happens, a family member feels that the advocate is counseling the patient in a self-destructive way, he or she should meet with the advocate and present the family viewpoint.

Review boards

Nowadays many jurisdictions have such boards composed of lawyers, psychiatrists, and lay people who review disputes between psychiatrists and patients. Commonly, these are cases in which the patient disputes the judgment of the psychiatrist with respect to dangerousness and involuntary hospitalization. The patient may also go to the review board to dispute the judgment of the psychiatrist with respect to incompetence to manage his financial affairs. The psychiatrist may approach the review board asking for permission to treat a competent patient against his will. This can be a particularly difficult situation on the psychiatric unit when a patient may present a threat, perhaps to other patients, but refuses to be treated. The law usually allows the psychiatrist to make interventions to 'control' the patient but not to 'treat' against his will. The review board process is a rather costly mechanism and extremely time-consuming. The boards tend to create an adversarial relationship between patient and doctor when a more collaborative relationship would work better. Patients' rights are important but the right to regain mental health is often omitted from the rhetoric of civil rights, and patients who successfully refuse treatment lose out by prolonging their psychotic state.

Conclusion

Most schizophrenic patients will require hospitalization at one time or another. The main reasons for hospitalization are serious risk to the patient or others around him and the need for close study and observation, including investigations. The first task is to secure the safety of the patient and others; then one tries to remove or at least reduce the active symptoms of illness. Hospitalization does not offer a permanent cure. Towards the end of the stay as the patient's condition normalizes, the main therapeutic emphasis is on initiating rehabilitative techniques that continue long after discharge.

THREE

Outpatient treatment

Treatment in hospital is only a fraction of total treatment since schizophrenia is potentially there for the rest of a person's life. About one-third of all individuals who suffer a first acute attack may never have another one. But for the other two-thirds, treatment may need to be lifelong. At this stage in medical knowledge, it is impossible to distinguish those who do from those who do not require long-term treatment. Because of this it is better to err on the safe side and to recommend outpatient treatment to everyone who has suffered an attack of schizophrenia.

In a hospital or clinic, patients are apt to have dealings with members of a treatment team as well as with other patients, some of them schizophrenic. In a private practice, the patient enters into a more exclusive relationship with his psychiatrist. In the former setting he may develop a degree of institutional reliance, in the latter a form of personal dependence. The tension between dependency and autonomy is a key issue in long-term treatment.

Outpatient visits

What gets accomplished
If an outpatient visits a clinic or hospital regularly, his doctor monitors his medications in order to prevent readmissions and

minimize drug side-effects. Virtually every patient will be on medication after an acute episode of schizophrenic illness. The patient engages in an active social program in order to counteract apathy and the tendency to withdraw. He learns progressively more about schizophrenia and to plan a rewarding life despite continuing symptoms of illness. Visits also enable him to benefit from individual, group, and family counseling about personal problems that may affect the illness. The patient takes advantage of liaison services with schools, jobs, housing authorities, training and financial assistance programs, and recreational facilities.

Who needs to come for outpatient visits?
Everyone who has been ill with schizophrenia needs treatment as an outpatient in order to prevent the return of the illness. This even includes people who consider themselves completely recovered since they, too, may be at risk. Making sure that the acute symptoms do not return usually means taking medication. Some people, in time, may find that they do not require medication. It is impossible, however, to predict in advance who these people will be. There needs to be a certain amount of trial and error to see who can do without it. A return of the original symptoms will mean that medication has to be continued. Needing medication is NOT a mark of weakness. It is a fact of life for the great majority of people with schizophrenia just as insulin is a fact of life for many people with diabetes.

A lack of energy and an aversion to being among people signal a need for outpatient treatment. The longer one isolates oneself after an acute bout of schizophrenia the harder it becomes to go out and face the world. Treatment provides occupational activity in areas of individual interest. It provides opportunities to meet people, opportunities to 'come out of the shell' in a gradual, non-pressured atmosphere with all the support that is necessary. Different programs do this in different ways.

Everyone who has had a schizophrenic illness needs to come to terms with what this means for the future. Many will need to have their relatives involved so that they, too, can learn about the illness and plan accordingly. Many will need help in educational, vocational, and occupational tasks – special school programs, for instance, or sheltered workshops.

How often do people need to attend?

Frequency of outpatient visits is an individual matter that depends on the patient's needs, the flexibility of the patient's and the therapist's hours, the nature and cost of the outpatient program, and the demands and the extent of the patient's other commitments. There is no ideal frequency. In general, however, visits become less frequent as time goes on. They may start as day care, when the patient is expected to attend daily for a major portion of the working day. Later there may be weekly visits, and eventually the intervals between visits may reach one, two, or three months.

Case manager

There has been a recent trend towards having a resource manager work with each schizophrenic patient on a long-term basis. This person may be from one of a variety of professional disciplines, such as occupational therapy, nursing, or social work. The case manager takes responsibility for all kinds of planning necessary for the patient. He will be involved in housing referrals, vocational planning and referrals, maintaining links with medical care and welfare services, and helping the patient negotiate with the important people in his life and cope with the stressors.

Outpatient treatment

Medication
See Chapter 4.

Maintenance of self-esteem
The best treatment for apathy and lack of interest is to bolster self-

confidence. This means opening windows on life through discussion, examination of self-defeating attitudes, gently applied pressure, and rewards for taking risks and trying new things. The treatment team provides the patient with a variety of nonthreatening opportunities to take up former interests and revamp old skills. The results of motivational work often seem to be better when the activities are carried out in a group setting, but this may not be so for everyone.

Therapies for daily activity

As a result of schizophrenia and hospitalization, many difficulties need to be overcome and new adjustments need to be made or life strategies developed. Many of the following kinds of therapy are used in outpatient treatment, although not necessarily all at the same time and not always in the same place:

- counseling or psychotherapy – individual and group – for the patient;
- education about schizophrenia, together with realistic planning for the future;
- counseling for interpersonal difficulties, in the form of marital therapy, family therapy, parenting groups, and other group therapies;
- vocational and educational assessment, counseling, and retraining;
- social therapies aimed at improved use of free time through various activities, such as sports, music, dancing, and art (all ways to become reinvolved in the world);
- teaching about and encouraging the development of self-help therapies (treatments that the patient administers himself) through assertiveness training, nutrition and hygiene clinics, social skills development, budget workshops, homemaking workshops;
- maintenance of liaison between the therapist or case manager in the mental health facility and a number of important people and agencies, such as the family, the family doctor, and the public health nurse; employment counselors and employer; sheltered

workshops, landlords, and group home supervisors; community activity centers; and self-help groups.

The role of the medical doctor
Any program for schizophrenia must have the active participation of a doctor. Schizophrenia is not merely a problem in living, it is first of all a medical disease. That is not to say that patients must be seen by doctors and by doctors only, but rather that doctors must be part of the program. A few family physicians are skilled in treating patients with schizophrenia. For the most part, however, psychiatrists who have both medical and psychiatric training are required from time to time.

Choice of medication and subsequent adjustment of dosage are skilled tasks which need constant monitoring. It is not enough simply to prescribe medication and then leave it at that. There must be frequent opportunities for reconsidering the dose and type of drug. Mental health professionals and paraprofessionals who are not doctors often, through experience, gain great expertise in monitoring medication. This happens, though, only in settings where psychiatrists are easily available for consultation. A discussion of medication appears in the next chapter; problems of long-term use are discussed on page 48.

Activity therapy
Programs must be able to counteract the apathy and social withdrawal associated with schizophrenia. Two elements are essential: a program that can occupy much of the patient's day; and a large enough group of helpers (including other patients) so that he does not feel alone with his disability, and so that a community can be established whose members begin to matter to each other.

Community links

An outpatient program for schizophrenia should be connected, by as many links as possible, to the community in which the person lives. In order to make effective use of these agencies when necessary, the therapeutic staff must be in continuing contact with the family, educational facilities; health facilities and medical personnel (family doctor, hospital clinic, dentists, dieticians) and exercise programs; vocational rehabilitation centers and employment agencies; government social agencies, residential facilities, community workers (public health nurses, police officers, community occupational therapists, visiting homemakers, mental health volunteers); sheltered workshops and graduated work programs; and leisure and social clubs for ex-mental patients. The more familiar the staff are with what is available in the community, the smoother the transition is for the recovering schizophrenic.

Whom to see for counseling

It makes sense for one person to be the primary therapist, counselor, or case manager and to act as program co-ordinator. This person need not be a doctor. The primary therapist can belong to any of the mental health professions or paraprofessions such as nursing, social work, psychology, rehabilitation, occupational therapy, and psychiatry, or, as in certain geographic regions, he may be the family doctor. Different aspects of the program will introduce the patient to other therapists who will be able to help in varying degrees. The primary therapist should be someone with whom the patient finds it easy to talk and to share problems. He need not be an expert in everything but must be understanding enough and knowledgeable enough to know when to link the schizophrenic and his family with other therapists and other therapeutic programs.

A time of distress for an outpatient often occurs when the primary therapist changes. Some programs use student trainees. This means frequent turnover when students graduate. Clients may feel disappointed by the recurrent changes; no sooner do they know a therapist than that therapist is on his way and they have to start all over again. For those not too overcome by the problem of separation, there are also a few advantages to changes in therapists. New therapists are often enthusiastic and their optimism is catching. In addition the helplessness of profound dependency is avoided by the change, and the patient is given the opportunity to learn how to form new relationships.

Are hospital-based programs best?

This question is controversial, and the answer depends on what is available in the community.

Hospitals have both advantages and disadvantages as settings for outpatient care. They are often familiar and trusted places for individuals who have attended the hospital as inpatients. A multidisciplinary team is usually available. Staff are familiar with medication problems. There is a pharmacy and the equipment necessary for intramuscular injections, should they be required. There is an emergency room for people with 'off-hours' problems and staff can usually be reached 24 hours a day. If hospitalization becomes necessary, the patient can be admitted to a place that is familiar and not intimidating.

However, attending a hospital seems to imply that one is still ill, rather than getting better. Going to hospital for treatment sounds more serious than attending a family doctor or a community program. Hospitals can be frightening places with bad memories for some people.

Community-based programs often have a more homelike atmosphere and, ideally, are housed in more spacious quarters than those available to outpatient departments. They are often situated in community centers that have gymnasiums, fields, and meeting rooms available for the use of participants. Some may include a sheltered work setting or a supervised residence. Some of the advantages of hospitals (availability of doctors, injection equipment, etc.) can be easily incorporated into community programs. These programs can function independently and not be subject to the various red-tape procedures of hospital clinics.

The treatment of schizophrenics by private practitioners is an important part of overall community care. It calls for a degree of selectivity on the part of the clinician since patients who are too disturbed, or who lack adequate social supports, are more effectively looked after in a clinic. Good communication between private practitioners and the hospital services allows for more effective crisis management and after-care planning.

Choosing a doctor

This is not an easy task. If you have a good physician, there is no need to look further. If, however, the doctor does not seem to know a great deal about schizophrenia or the drugs used in treatment, or if he is always busy and uninterested, then it would be wise to seek out someone else. The best way to find out who in your area is good in this field is to talk to people who have schizophrenia, or to their families.

Choosing a program

During the rehabilitation period, the patient may have many opportunities to attend different programs. It is worthwhile to inspect various programs, looking at the physical facilities and meeting the significant staff. It is very important when one is schizophrenic to be an informed consumer. Some programs are very good indeed but quite unsuitable for a particular patient because of the nature of the patients who are currently there, the degree of strictness of the rules and regulations, or the distance from his home. All of these factors need to be borne in mind.

Does supportive treatment need to continue forever?

In some form, it probably does, although support needs vary from individual to individual.

People who have had serious health problems, and schizophrenia is a case in point, should always have easy and immediate access to health counseling. Being in treatment does not mean that the frequency of contact should continue forever as in the first few years following hospitalization. Staying in touch, perhaps by telephone only, may be sufficient as time goes by. The ex-patient should always have someone whom he can call in an emergency. If the primary therapist leaves, the ex-patient should arrange to be linked to someone else, even though all troublesome symptoms may have disappeared long before.

How to recognize the reappearance of illness

Schizophrenic illness has characteristic early signs and recurrent patterns, even though some people say that the original schizophrenic illness came without warning, 'out of the blue.' After the first episode, however, people have been sensitized and are more able to recognize early warning signs, even though the signs may be slow to develop and vague in nature.

Each individual has his own set of early warning signs. Some frequently encountered ones are: diminished ability to concentrate, increased irritability, uncontrollable moods, increased self-consciousness, difficulties in thinking, social withdrawal, increasing suspicion of other people's motives, inability to sleep.

It is important to recognize one's own early signs of illness and to be able to connect them with a trigger. The trigger is very often overstimulation in its various forms, but it may also be other psychological stresses (loss of support, disappointment, rejection) or physical stresses (exhaustion, fever, alcohol, drugs). Too many life changes too quickly can precipitate acute illness. Major life changes, if they can be controlled, are best spaced far apart.

Case vignette
One patient, who has never been hospitalized for schizophrenia, takes a very small amount of neuroleptics which keep all her

symptoms at bay. In her case, an early sign that trouble is brewing is headache. Whenever she feels this particularly severe headache, she doubles up on her medication and is back to normal in a week.

How to control acute illness

Control consists of removing the trigger and increasing medication.

Recognized early, the progression of illness can be stopped by temporarily increasing the dose of medication and temporarily withdrawing from what has become an overstimulating environment. The person with schizophrenia has to learn to avoid overstimulation. At the same time he must avoid understimulation, which leads to apathy and lack of initiative. This balancing act is difficult but can be learned. When acute symptoms begin to develop, it is usually a sign that work pressure must be eased, personal relationships soft-pedaled, expectations lowered, and the schedule of activities slowed. These measures, when promptly initiated, can frequently prevent hospital admission. They are, of course, *temporary* measures to be discontinued when the crisis has passed.

Are vitamins useful?

They are not useful for schizophrenia. Most doctors feel that if diet is adequate extra vitamins are unnecessary. Large-dose vitamins (megavitamins) have been claimed to be useful in treating schizophrenia, but carefully controlled studies fail to support this claim. There is no question that some people do improve, however, while taking vitamins. It may be that the improvement is due to the neuroleptic drugs they are taking at the same time; it may be that their condition is not schizophrenia; or it may be that the patient belongs to that 30 percent who recover anyway and stay well. Alternatively, the structure and effort involved in maintaining the vitamin intake may be therapeutic. And, of course, believing in the efficacy of a therapy and the therapist is therapeutic in itself.

Are special diets necessary?

Nutrition is important to well-being but this is no more true for the person with schizophrenia than for any other individual. The general apathy that often follows schizophrenia means that little interest is taken in anything, including food. If this leads to poor nutrition, fatigue and lack of energy may well increase. This is a special problem for people living alone who do not have the motivation to prepare proper meals. A well-balanced diet should be encouraged but special diets are not necessary. Some special diets may in fact be harmful if essential ingredients of a regular diet are missing. Many people would rather follow a diet than take medicines, and special diets for schizophrenia are frequently popularized in the press. In the last few years gluten-free diets, low-sugar diets, liquid-only diets, milk-free diets, and periodic fasts have been hailed as the 'cure' for schizophrenia. These fads have no merit whatsoever.

Medication for schizophrenia may lead to undesired weight gain. Starvation diets and appetite suppressants are *not* the answer. The physician should be consulted for better solutions.

How safe are 'new' therapies?

It is best not to discontinue treatment that is 'tried and true' in favor of intriguing but as yet untested alternatives. Since there is still no 'total answer' to schizophrenia, people tend to expect too much from any new discovery as it comes along. This is a form of wishful thinking. New discoveries are steps towards the goal of understanding the disease, but each one is only a partial answer to the many problems involved. Going from doctor to doctor, city to city, looking for a miracle cure is a frustrating and ineffective way of looking after oneself.

Is psychotherapy useful?

Since psychological events on their own do not – as far as we know – cause schizophrenia, it is unlikely that psychological treatment on its own can cure it. However, getting to know oneself better, understanding the nature of one's problems, recognizing one's feelings, exploring one's reactions, and planning ahead realistically are all important. Psychotherapy that promotes these activities is very useful in schizophrenia. It is not intended as a cure but as an approach to self-understanding and towards understanding events in the immediate environment which may precipitate a relapse.

Psychotherapy can be carried out between two individuals, in a group, or in a family. One form of psychotherapy may be more useful at one time; another may be preferred at another time. The use of medication does not preclude psychotherapy.

What are the dangers of alcohol and street drugs?

Some substances (alcohol, marijuana) have an immediate, relaxing effect that is first experienced as soothing, but they may have a later effect that is harmful.

Amphetamines and hallucinogens (also marijuana, hashish) can trigger episodes of schizophrenia and should not be used. Certain cold tablets, weight-reducing pills, or even nose drops can precipitate episodes of illness. Patients can learn to be alert to the effect of chemical substances (and even foods such as coffee or spices) on their individual symptoms. Alcohol is also known to increase the side-effects of neuroleptics, both parkinsonism and sedation.

Case vignette
A 45-year-old male patient has had a relatively successful life (marriage, children, steady employment, artistic accomplishments) but has had four very severe schizophrenic breakdowns all of which almost led to death because of the risks to which he exposed himself during these disorganized periods. In all four instances,

these breakdowns were triggered by marijuana use. When not smoking marijuana he has never experienced schizophrenic symptoms.

Are self-help groups useful?

Organizations set up by patients for mutual support have been around for many years (for example, Recovery; Grow) and have played an important role in helping ex-patients readjust to society. More recently there has been increased development of groups concerned with patients' rights that have looked at psychiatry from the vantage point of the 'consumer' and have found the psychiatric profession wanting. There are still controversial areas of treatment of schizophrenia and other illnesses, and even when the best treatment is prescribed its application may not always be carried out in the most humane manner. It is crucial that those who work in psychiatry pay careful attention to the criticisms of the consumers.

Naturally the people most likely to join patients' rights groups are those who personally feel they have been mistreated. There is a danger in such groups of developing a polarized attitude, condemning a particular mode of treatment generally, whereas the treatment itself may be fine but the particular use of it inappropriate. For example, Judi Chamberlin has written a book, *On Our Own*, that has many important things to say about mental patients' associations but which categorically rejects medication: 'Drugs, euphemistically called psychiatric medication, are given to patients with the avowed purpose of changing their "sick" thoughts, and the process is called treatment.' Her book was described as 'an honest and intelligent assault on psychiatric atrocities' by the psychiatrist Thomas Szasz, who rejects the commonly held view of schizophrenia as an illness of the brain. Contrast this with the book *Psychobattery* by Theresa Spitzer. It too is a criticism of psychiatry and psychiatrists, but attacks the use of psychotherapy in situations where medication is indicated. Both these books make valuable points as long as they are not taken to mean that all medication or all psychotherapy should be discarded.

Ideally there should exist a mutually beneficial relationship between patients' rights groups and professionals, each with an open approach, willing to listen and to learn from one another. (See Appendix II for a list of self-help groups.)

Confidentiality of information

Legally and ethically, no information about a patient can be shared outside a treatment team without the patient's written consent. This rule applies even when the person asking for information is obviously asking for the patient's good. In other words, even if a lawyer who wants to defend a patient requires medical information to prove his client innocent, that, too, cannot be given without the patient's written consent. If a mother or father or spouse wants information that might make it easier and better for them to deal with the patient at home, that, too, cannot be given without consent. Often mental health staff appear distant and secretive to relatives because they are concerned about not revealing confidential information. Relatives and staff need to understand the need for knowledge, on the one hand, and the need to preserve confidences, on the other.

By the same token, relatives sometimes want to tell mental health staff about the patient's behavior but want this information to be kept secret. They may find some therapists unwilling to listen to this type of confidential information because knowledge of facts is not judged useful unless its source can be discussed openly with the patient. If the relative does not want the patient to know where the information came from, then the information itself may be of little use. Therapists need to appreciate that many relatives need help and support to deal with this problem. The most helpful way is for the relative to come to the therapist with the patient to discuss the troublesome behavior openly.

Access to the clinical record

Only the treating team has access to a person's clinical record.

No one else can look at the clinical record without the written consent of the patient. The only exception to this is that researchers are sometimes given permission to study all the charts of people who, for instance, were admitted to hospital on a certain day or who share a common diagnosis or who are being treated with the same medication. Research to further medical understanding is usually part of a university hospital setting and is always under the strict supervision of the hospital or university ethical review board. Any information recorded for research purposes is coded by number; the patient's name does not appear on the research data. If patients are interested in seeing parts of their own clinical record, they should discuss their concerns with their doctor. Different jurisdictions have different regulations on accessibility of medical records.

Dissatisfaction with outpatient treatment

Dissatisfaction usually has to do with one or more of the following: the patient is not getting better; he suffers from side-effects of medication; he feels a lack of interest on the part of the therapist; the therapist is unavailable at a critical time; the therapist and patient (or relative) have different philosophies of treatment.

All these require discussion with the therapist. Usually satisfactory solutions can be found. If, after discussion, no resolution is found, the patient or family is justified in asking for a second opinion or arranging for referral to another therapist. This can usually be done through the family doctor.

If the patient begins treatment with a new therapist, it is important for the new therapist to have as accurate a picture as possible of the patient's prior illness. Otherwise, an inaccurate diagnosis may be made, and an inappropriate treatment plan may be put into effect.

FOUR

Medications

Introduction

Individuals with schizophrenia, and their families, sometimes find the array of different medicines used in schizophrenia bewildering. They find it hard to sort out which medicines do what.

In other chapters of this book, whenever we refer to 'medication,' we mean neuroleptics, which are anti-schizophrenic agents. Whenever we mention 'staying on medication,' 'increasing or decreasing medication,' or 'stopping medication,' we are referring to neuroleptics.

Other kinds of medicines are also used at times in the course of a schizophrenic illness: pills used for neuromuscular side-effects of neuroleptics, anxiolytics, mood stabilizers, and antidepressants. These will also be briefly discussed in this chapter.

Neuroleptics

Neuroleptics are drugs that reverse psychotic symptoms. They used to be called major tranquilizers, but that name is not much used now because it is misleading. Some of them do 'tranquilize,' but not all, and the tranquilization or sedation is a side-effect, not the effect for which they are prescribed. (Tranquilization is more a property of the so-called minor tranquilizers or anxiolytics. These agents are *not* neuroleptics, nor are they related chemically to the neuroleptics.)

There are about 20 neuroleptics in common use and each has several names. One name is the officially approved name and the others are 'trade names' – each drug company gives its own brand name to the drug. In this chapter we shall use the official name. Appendix III includes the trade names. Often the same chemical formula produced by different companies is priced differently. Sometimes a 100-milligram tablet, say, costs quite a bit less than two 50-milligram tablets. It is wise to price the tablets in the pharmacy and to discuss price and all other questions about medication with the prescribing doctor as well as with the pharmacist.

The neuroleptics come in many different chemical structures. They all, however, act in the *same* way in schizophrenia. They all reduce the transmission of the brain chemical dopamine, which carries a message from certain brain cells to others. The reduction of dopamine transmission results in fewer hallucinations and delusions and less illogical thinking. The exact progress is unknown, but it has something to do with the nature of the nerve pathways that are under the control of the dopamine molecule. All neuroleptic molecules can assume the shape of a dopamine molecule; in this way they 'fool' the receptor for dopamine from getting through and firing the cell. Neuroleptics work well for schizophrenia and for a few related disorders.

Although all neuroleptics interfere with dopamine in the same way, they each have different properties otherwise. For instance, they differ in their effects on brain chemicals other than dopamine. (See Appendix III.) Chlorpromazine, for example, interferes with noradrenaline transmission and may consequently be quite sedating. Thioridazine affects acetylcholine transmission and this may produce unwanted effects such as blurring of vision, dry mouth, and, in the male, problems with erection and ejaculation. Interference with acetylcholine transmission, however, can be useful because the brain maintains a balance between dopamine and acetylcholine. When the level of one decreases, there is a relative increase in the other. So with most neuroleptics, the level of dopamine drops and there is a relative upsurge of acetylcholine. This can cause tremor, muscle stiffness, muscle spasm, and motor restlessness. Thioridazine has the advantage of not producing these muscle effects because it interferes with acetylcholine as much as it does with dopamine. But, especially in older people, anticholinergic effects may be harmful. Thioridazine has to be used very carefully, especially when given in high doses.

Neuroleptics such as perphenazine, trifluoperazine, fluphenazine, and haloperidol dissolve easily in fat tissue and therefore easily penetrate nerve membranes. For this reason they can be effective in small doses. Seven milligrams of haloperidol may have the same antipsychotic potency as 100 milligrams of chlorpromazine or thioridazine. Relatives often wonder why one person has to take so many milligrams of a drug while another takes such a seemingly small amount. In fact, the person on the smaller dose may be taking a 'stronger' antipsychotic drug. Patients often wonder why they seem to have so many side-effects and other patients do not, why one seems to improve so rapidly almost as soon as a medicine is started, and another takes so long to improve. That is because each person responds differently, and the type and dose of medication have to be individually tailored.

The type and dose of a neuroleptic that a person will respond to depend on many factors such as height and weight, activity, diet, physical health, other pills being taken at the same time, speed of digestion, and extent of body fat stores. It is hard to predict exactly which neuroleptic a given person will respond to.

Sometimes *depot* or long-acting medicines are used. These are neuroleptics given to last for a week or several weeks at a time. They are given by injection, deep into the muscle. Fluphenazine decanoate, flupenthixol, pipotiazine, fluspirilene, and haloperidol decanoate are commonly used depot drugs. The advantage of this treatment for people who are poor absorbers is that it bypasses the digestive tract. It costs less. It is easier to keep track of, and patients do not have to rely on memory in order to take their pills as prescribed. The patient comes once a week (or less often) to the clinic for his injection and, while there, may also take part in other clinic activities. If a patient on depot medication stops taking it, his nurse and doctor are immediately aware of the fact. Many patients, however, prefer to take treatment actively rather than passively at the hands of somebody else. Some patients, though relatively few, are able to self-administer depot medication.

Drug refusal

It is very common for patients at some time to stop taking their medication. This happens sooner or later with most patients. The reason will vary from one patient to another. Some common reasons include:
- the nuisance of having to take medication on a regular basis;
- the tendency of patients to convince themselves that they are in fact not ill;
- the avoidance of unpleasant drug side-effects;
- a rejection of the pill which is a constant reminder that they have an illness;
- a misunderstanding of schizophrenia, thinking that it can be conquered by willpower alone;
- a reflection of low self-esteem and an unconscious wish to sabotage improvement;
- fear of the long-term effects of the drugs.
There may be other explanations as well. This kind of refusal is a major cause of concern for those who care about the patient and for those who are trying to treat him. What can be very disheartening for all concerned is that many patients stop their medication repeatedly despite frightening consequences. When somebody stops medication the relapse may occur within a few days, though it usually takes many weeks and can take as long as a year or two. The longer the relapse-free interval, the greater the likelihood that

maintenance drugs may not be needed; but the trial needs to be under medical supervision. It is important for everybody concerned about the person to urge him to resume his treatment. The patient needs to be educated about the effects of the medication, including its usefulness in preventing psychotic recurrence. Staff and family need to try to find out why medication was stopped and to try to help patients to deal with their feelings and concerns in this area. Sometimes all that one can do is stand by. The hope is that the patient will learn by the consequences he experiences.

Many residences for psychiatric patients make medication adherence a condition of living in them. Some families learn to do this as well. In other words, they allow their son or daughter to live at home only if medication is regularly taken. A firm stance on this important issue prevents much heartache and potential harm.

Long-term effects

Many patients worry about the long-term effects of medicines. Neuroleptics have now been in use for 39 years, so it is unlikely that anything new, as far as dangerous long-term effects go, will be discovered now. Some long-term effects do exist. A few people, after many years of using neuroleptics, develop skin discoloration and some opaque deposits in the cornea or lens of the eye. These do not interfere with vision. More people, after years of use, develop tics and spasms of muscles, especially the muscles around the face. In many cases, when the neuroleptics are stopped, these tics and spasms initially get a little worse but then disappear. In some people, though, especially older people, they do not disappear even after the neuroleptics have been stopped for some time. The reason for this is not clear. Families may find these tics difficult to accept although the patients do not seem aware of them and often feel they are a small price to pay for the security of staying free of psychosis. Tics and tremors that persist after medication is stopped are called *tardive dyskinesia*, which means late-appearing disjointed movements. All the commonly used antipsychotics can produce tardive dyskinesia if used over a period of time. In a minority of patients these movements can involve large muscles of the trunk and can even interfere with breathing. From time to time there are patients who are particularly vulnerable to this dyskinesia and who develop it in severe form within a relatively short time span. Drug companies are trying to synthesize new drugs that will not cause this unfortunate side-effect. Doctors are trying various strategies of prescribing these medications in an effort to reduce the risk of tardive dyskinesia. What appears to work best is to keep neuroleptic doses as low as possible for any particular individual. Patients and families need also to be aware of the paradox of tardive dyskinesia. When the dose is raised, the dyskinetic movements actually are reduced, at least for a time. In cases of severe dyskinesia, this strategy must sometimes be adopted.

When to stop medication

Many relatives ask: 'When should medication be stopped?' No one really knows the answer to this question. Some individuals, even though they continue to have schizophrenic symptoms, can stop their pills without the symptoms getting worse. Other individuals, though, may be free of all symptoms and feel healthy, but when the pills are stopped they once again develop a full-fledged schizophrenic attack. This unpredictability is what makes the decision about when to stop neuroleptics so difficult. Many doctors advocate a gradual reduction with close observation and reporting on subjective feelings. Some patients get to know themselves so well that they can tell when symptoms are about to develop and can then, on their own, take extra medication. It usually takes many years, though, before this can be done well. Occasionally doctors recommend drug holidays – periods of time without medication – but for most people this is too risky. It can be misleading to stop medication because, though feeling subjectively better for a time, one is at risk for another serious breakdown in the future. It is wise to follow the doctor's advice very faithfully on this and all other issues related to the taking of medication, although it is also wise to keep informed and ask for second opinions if doubts arise.

Pills for neuromuscular side-effects (antiparkinsonians)

Since there is a balance in the brain between the neurotransmitters dopamine and acetylcholine, the use of neuroleptics to block dopamine frequently produces a relative preponderance of acetylcholine. This leads to a state that looks like Parkinson's disease: tremor, rigidity, restlessness, expressionless face, and, sometimes, muscle spasms. These side-effects are often short-lived and are usually reversible by the addition of 'anticholinergic' agents, commonly called *side-effect pills* or *antiparkinsonian pills*. There are many of these. Perhaps the most commonly prescribed ones are benztropine (Cogentin), trihexyphenidyl (Artane), and procyclidine (Kemadrin). These are not given for the symptoms of schizophrenia or for the prevention of relapse but for side-effects of neuroleptics. If the patient is not taking neuroleptics, he does not need to take these pills. If he is still taking neuroleptics but, as is usual, the initial muscular side-effects have disappeared, the side-effect pills may be discontinued or taken only as needed. On their own these pills are potentially toxic drugs and may produce their own side-effects. Some muscle side-effects respond better to one type of pill and some to another. If side-effect control is not satisfactory, let the doctor know. Some side-effects, such as inner restlessness, are mainly subjective so that only the patient is aware of them. The patient needs to be schooled to recognize these effects and to report them, and doctors must be schooled to listen attentively to the patient's complaints.

Anxiolytics

Although several kinds of drugs may be effective in reducing anxiety, the benzodiazepines are used most often because they work well and are very safe. There are quite a few benzodiazepines in common use, the best known probably being diazepam. They are distinguished most by their duration of action, acting quickly but for short periods, others having delayed onset times but being effective for a longer duration. The shorter-acting benzodiazepines are best for anxiety; the longer-acting ones are best for nighttime sedation.

In addition to quieting anxiety and inducing sleep, the benzodiazepines also have anticonvulsant properties and are good muscle relaxants. In schizophrenia they may be used for fear and anxiety, trouble sleeping, or muscle tension, or, sometimes, to raise the convulsion threshold, which is lowered by neuroleptics. What that means is that for people who are prone to epileptic seizures, neuroleptics may sometimes make them more prone. In that case neuroleptics may be combined with benzodiazepines. The neuroleptic-benzodiazepine combination also works well in people who are made restless by the neuroleptics or whose muscles tend to tense up as a side-effect of neuroleptics. The use of benzodiazepines with neuroleptics at night for sleep or in the day to reduce anxiety can help to lower the dose of neuroleptics and to make treatment safer and freer of unpleasant side-effects.

Benzodiazepines can lead to sedation and to clouding of memory. Tolerance to them can develop and a psychological dependency on them can become established in some long-term users. In general, however, properly prescribed, these drugs are a useful adjunct to neuroleptics in the treatment of schizophrenia, and they are extremely safe. One reason why they might be contraindicated in some patients is that they can be disinhibiting. They can make it harder to control or resist harmful impulses. For this reason they may not be in the best interests of some schizophrenic patients.

They work by binding to benzodiazepine receptors in the brain. These receptors exist in the cortex of the brain, the site of the anticonvulsant effect. They exist in other parts of the brain called the amygdala and the hippocampus. It is here that the anti-anxiety effect is thought to originate. They also exist in the spinal cord, and this is the site of the muscle-relaxing effects.

Benzodiazepines exert effects on brain neurotransmitters. Most especially they appear to potentiate or increase the natural effect of gamma-amino-butyric acid (GABA). This neurotransmitter inhibits the firing of nerve cells or slows down brain excitability. Benzodiazepines put a further brake on this slowdown – an effect which is very welcome to a person in an overagitated state.

Anticonvulsants

Besides the benzodiazepines, conventional anticonvulsants like phenytoin may sometimes be used to raise the convulsive threshold. A more common anticonvulsant that is receiving attention in schizophrenia and in affective disorders is carbamazepine. It seems to reduce impulsivity and to equalize mood. Some schizophrenics may respond better to it than to neuroleptics. Unfortunately, it can have toxic effects and regular blood tests may be required.

Lithium salts

Lithium is a mood stabilizer and requires regular blood tests to ensure proper blood levels. Lithium is used more in affective disorders than in schizophrenia, but it may be added to a neuroleptic regimen to counteract depression, improve impulsivity, or prevent mood swings. Neuroleptic-lithium combinations may produce more side-effects than treatment with one class of drug alone, so people on such combinations require extra-careful monitoring.

Antidepressants

There are many antidepressants. The most common ones are called *tricyclics*, because of their three-ring chemical structure. They are thought to exert their action by controlling the brain chemicals known as noradrenaline and serotonin. The best known are imipramine and amitriptyline. They are used for depression and may be used in schizophrenia when there is a secondary depression present, or in schizo-affective schizophrenia. They have side-effects of their own and may add to the effects of neuroleptics and antiparkinsonians, so dosages of all three need to be carefully adjusted. Antidepressants take about 10 days to three weeks to start working, so one must not expect depressive symptoms to respond right away. Doses often need to be raised in a gradual, stepwise fashion before the best effects are obtained. Like neuroleptics they are usually best taken once every night. Sometimes two or three different antidepressants have to be tried before the right one is found.

Other medications

Other medications (antihistamines, propranolol, hypnotics) are sometimes used for individuals with special difficulties, and, of course, new agents are continually being developed. Do not hesitate to ask the doctor to explain the use of any medications with which you are not familiar. Amphetamines and related substances used in weight-reducing tablets are not advisable for schizophrenics. They may trigger symptoms of psychosis. It is important to make certain that *all* prescribing doctors know *all* the medications a person is taking, including aspirins, nose drops, eye drops, contraceptive pills, allergy shots, vitamins, and such chemicals as caffeine (coffee, tea, cocoa, cola drinks), alcohol, marijuana, and nicotine. Caffeine makes neuroleptic side-effects much worse and also intensifies anxiety. Medication, especially in combination with other chemicals, can lead to drowsiness, so driving or exposure to dangerous machinery must be avoided until the drug schedule is well established.

FIVE

How relatives can help

Introduction

Relatives usually want to help the patient but feel helpless. They are not sure about the right way to help. Different authorities give them contradictory advice. When they get involved, they may be told they are overinvolved. When they back off, they may be told they are uninterested. In fact, there is no *one* right way. A particular solution may work with one person at one time but not another, or not with the same person the next time around. Much of what follows is advice rather than foolproof prescription. Try one way, give it time, and see what happens. If it seems to be working, continue it. If it seems not to be working, try another tack. Speak to your relative's therapists – they may have some good suggestions. Above all, don't give up. Through much trial and error a workable solution will eventually be found.

When a person seems disturbed

Usually relatives have no idea what is wrong when a family member becomes ill with schizophrenia for the first time. If the person lives with the family, they may have noticed some strange behavior. Not knowing how to explain it, they may attribute it to a 'phase,' not unlike what they themselves or others in the family have experienced in the past. If the behavior continues to be decidedly 'odd,' the family will wonder about bad companions and drink or drugs. All sorts of explanations will be considered, the possibility of illness usually being left to the last.

Perhaps the first thing a family can do, then, is to consider mental illness when unexplained behavior transforms someone you love into a stranger. Information about mental illnesses can be obtained from libraries, mental health associations, family doctors, psychiatrists, and psychiatric hospitals. Once mental illness is suspected, a number of steps can be taken.

The family must make every effort to speak with the individual concerned and to ask him what he thinks is happening. He may well be more worried and frightened than the family. He may already have recognized that something very puzzling has happened to his mind, to his emotions, and, it may seem to him, to the world.

The family should encourage him to see his family physician. General health problems can sometimes lead to the appearance of psychiatric symptoms. For example, disorders of the thyroid gland or of the adrenal gland produce emotional disturbances. A full physical checkup is always indicated.

The family needs to consult long and seriously with the physician about the most likely diagnosis. The physician may not be sure and may suggest referral to a psychiatrist. This is not as ominous as it may sound at first. The psychiatrist may reassure the family that this is not schizophrenia. Or he may feel it is a mild form of the illness that can be treated in an outpatient setting.

Schizophrenia is a potentially serious condition and the diagnosis should not be made lightly. All concerned will want to ensure that it is correctly made. A period of hospitalization may therefore be essential for proper diagnosis. While an inpatient on a ward, a person enters into many relationships and is confronted with numerous tasks. During all of these he reveals himself increasingly to those around him, especially to his doctor and nurse. This is the type of intensive assessment that is difficult to carry out on an outpatient basis. The patient will, predictably, not want admission. The family can be of great assistance by being informed and informative about hospital routines, and by being reassuring and consistently supportive of the decision to admit (see Chapter 2, on inpatient treatment).

When the patient is in hospital

Regular visits are usually appreciated and most psychiatric units have liberal visiting policies. Visiting may be restricted during meeting times, therapy hours, and meals. The ward staff will advise the patient and his family on what specific items might be needed for the stay in hospital.

The relatives are often the only people who can supply the important facts about what led up to the current symptoms, and their story is very important for diagnosis. The patient is often too frightened and perplexed to give a coherent story. Hospital staff ask the relatives to give their version of recent happenings to complement the patient's account. The following is an example of how essential it is for the psychiatric staff to interview the family:

The patient was a 20-year-old male Portuguese immigrant. He entered the hospital terror-stricken and it was hard to obtain his story. It finally was learned that he had broken up with his girlfriend in the recent past and heard voices in his head saying he was a homosexual. The voices told him to visit a psychic in order to obtain a magic potion to cure him. He followed the instructions and consulted with the psychic but did not have enough money to pay her what she asked. Because of this, she told him, he said, that she would follow him and kill him. The story sounded so bizarre and implausible and the man was so frightened and disorganized that a tentative diagnosis of schizophrenia was made. The auditory hallucinations seemed to bear it out.

When the parents were interviewed with the help of an interpreter, they gave some very helpful background material. They said their son moped about for months after being rejected by his girlfriend. He was not interested in any other girls so his brothers and his friends, in order to 'get him out of it,' teased him about being a homosexual. Apparently this was a common tease in their community but their son was particularly sensitive to it because he was rather short and had always thought he looked 'too girlish.' In their community it was the custom to visit psychics and obtain special potions, no matter what the ailment. The mother was herself in treatment by a psychic for 'rheumatism.' It was also true that psychics often charged very high fees, especially if they thought the ailment was of so embarrassing a nature that the client would not complain. Threats of revenge were not unheard of. In other words, all of the son's fears made sense in context. His emotions and behaviors no longer appeared to fit the diagnosis of schizophrenia. In fact he recovered very quickly, especially after his ex-girlfriend came to visit.

When the patient leaves hospital

After receiving a diagnosis of schizophrenia both patient and family may feel deflated and hopeless. It is important for all concerned to realize that although there are serious implications, everyday functioning need not be interfered with in schizophrenia. One does not usually speak about 'cure' in schizophrenia, since symptoms do come back or may come back. One speaks, instead, of 'social recovery,' meaning functioning well in all areas of life (educational, vocational, recreational, interpersonal) as long as treatment is continued. In this schizophrenia is not different from many other medical conditions: diabetes, asthma, arthritis. When these illnesses strike in young adulthood, they disrupt many areas of functioning at first. With proper and ongoing treatment, the victim of schizophrenia is usually able to carry on with his life as before. Recovery, however, may be slow and, in some instances, incomplete.

When recovery is not complete, it may be difficult for the individual and for the family to accept limitations on what is possible. In the beginning it may be very hard to give up long-dreamed-of plans. A university education, for instance, may need to be abandoned. Marriage and a family may be unrealistic. The goal has to be self-sufficiency for the individual and that may mean a total turnaround in terms of previous vocational aspirations.

The most important thing a relative can do is to let the person concerned know that there is a future for him and that he, the relative, sees it as a rewarding future, far though it may be from what was originally hoped for. This message can be conveyed in many ways. Talk to him and show an interest in what he is doing as part of his treatment program. Be enthusiastic about what he is doing even though at first it may sound dull and repetitious to you. Do not let your own standards of what is menial work and what is rewarding work erode your enthusiasm. Routine, predictable, nonstressful tasks are important for the schizophrenic to master first.

What to do about not taking medication

For most people with schizophrenia, continuing medication is the basis of staying well and must be established as an easy-to-follow routine. Do not passively accept drug refusal. Insist that the patient discuss this crucial issue with the psychiatrist.

What about drug abusers

Street drugs and schizophrenia do not mix. This message must be reinforced by family and friends.

Should a schizophrenic be pushed?

Even before getting a job, the individual must become self-sufficient in looking after personal hygiene, meals, and clothes. Relatives can help by expecting and encouraging him to master self-care tasks. How much to push depends on the particular stages of illness and on what one is pressing the schizophrenic person to do.

When full social recovery has taken place and the condition is stable, the schizophrenic should be treated like any other family member. He should be expected to assume full responsibility for himself and take part in the duties of the household to the same degree as others.

When there are clear signs of continuing illness, the family must decide what is most important and what is less so. For instance, if he continues to have many active symptoms of schizophrenia, then ensuring that he takes his medication regularly is more important than encouraging him to make his bed. Making sure that he attends treatment appointments has to come before visiting friends. Sometimes, in their zeal to have everything return to normal as quickly as possible, relatives expect too much too soon. It is usually more successful to decide what is crucial and make sure that *that* gets done. The rest can wait.

The most difficult time to decide whether to push or not is the in-between stage when the individual is better than he was but not as well as he might be. Probably the easiest way to start is by expecting him to do the tasks he enjoys. That guarantees success, and small successes increase enjoyment and feelings of self-worth. The household tasks that he dislikes can be left undone for the time being. It is best when the whole family agrees to this so that envy and jealousy do not develop. If the schizophrenic family member prefers putting out garbage to washing the dishes, he can forgo his turn at the dishes and make it up by an extra turn at the garbage. When you run out of enjoyable tasks, the next easiest to do are the simple routines. The convalescent schizophrenic patient is often too preoccupied to think things out. Giving him a long list of complicated instructions does not work. Ask him to do *one* thing at a time. Routines are easier to follow than constantly changing demands. Do not hesitate to speak to him and to his therapist about what is appropriate as far as demands go and about what is too little, or too much.

When to leave the recovering schizophrenic alone at home

Everyone needs a break at times, especially if the home situation is tense and stressful. Individuals with schizophrenia will not always welcome the temporary departure of someone they care about, but that is not a reason to stay constantly at home.

It makes sense to stay at home when the schizophrenic is ill and not able to care for himself. When he is well and stable there is no reason not to go out for the evening, away for weekends, or away for a long vacation. The most difficult time to decide is when he is clearly not as ill as he was but is not yet fully himself. In such cases, relatives often stay at home because they feel too badly about leaving their charge to 'fend for himself.' A wiser move would be to prepare him well in advance; make the necessary arrangements for adequate supervision; inform relatives, neighbors, and therapist; and go on vacation. It will be good for you and good practice for the schizophrenic in his pursuit of self-sufficiency.

Holidays for the patient

If the recovering schizophrenic wants to take a holiday away from home, what then? The first such venture is very anxiety-provoking for the family. The best advice is to let him go provided his illness is stabilized. Try to help him make appropriate plans. Help him make contingency plans in case the original ones fall through. Stand by him whether the trip succeeds or not. Becoming self-sufficient involves trials and errors. The errors cannot be avoided. In fact, they are essential to eventual success.

Always make sure that adequate amounts of medication are taken along on the trip. For long absences, a statement from the doctor about the type and dose of medication should always accompany the patient. If the trip is to a sunny climate make sure the patient has an appropriate sun-screen lotion. Many lotions contain para-amino benzoic acid (PABA) that protects skin sensitized by neuroleptic medication against ultraviolet light. PABA, however, is quite allergenic and non-PABA containing sun-screens are also available.

Should the schizophrenic socialize?

When an opportunity to socialize comes up, the individual should decide what he prefers to do about it. A big difficulty for relatives has to do with the schizophrenic's 'ambivalence.' This means that he frequently cannot make up his mind about what he prefers. Asked what he wants to do, he says one thing and then does another. This can drive the family to despair. It is important to remember that the schizophrenic is not doing this on purpose. He is literally unable to make up his mind. If this happens, the family has to be decisive. They can, for instance, flip a coin and then insist that the course of action be dictated by the results of the coin toss. They can call a family vote and insist that the majority vote decides. The patient is usually grateful if he is helped with decision-making in an impartial, nonautocratic manner.

Sometimes the schizophrenic family member wants to accompany the family on a visit, but the others are reluctant to take him because of his potentially embarrassing behavior. He may be afraid of eating in public or meeting new people, or he may experience perplexity or panic. Socially unacceptable behavior is likely to vary with anxiety. The more comfortable a person feels, the more likely he is to behave well. Try taking him first to close friends. Discuss with him afterwards any socially unacceptable behavior that occurs and try, together, to figure out how it could have been avoided. It is usually worthwhile to experiment. Visits that promise to be embarrassing often turn out to be thoroughly enjoyable. There will, of course, be times when it will not be appropriate to take the patient. For example, a schizophrenic who has an overpowering fear of eating in public would make a poor guest at a banquet. The family's right and need for privacy must also be respected.

As the ex-patient gains confidence, he should be encouraged to plan his own entertainment. Recontacting old friends can be an ordeal for many reasons. Frequently the presence of a serious illness has destroyed what was once a close friendship. Patients may be more comfortable, at first, associating with new acquaintances whom they met in hospital. They share a bond of common experience that makes communication easier. Relatives often do not approve of these new friends who may be from the wrong social circle. It is important to remember that friendships may present difficulties for schizophrenics and that most attempts at socialization should be encouraged.

How to treat the schizophrenic

When a person has socially recovered, he should be treated like anyone else in the family. Until then allowances may have to be made. The schizophrenic, however, is not the only person in the family, and it is not realistic to treat him as if he were. The needs and feelings of other family members must also be considered. Social recovery can take some time. Meanwhile the schizophrenic may be preferentially treated. For example, he may be relieved of chores he is unable to do. This can be annoying to others, especially to his brothers and sisters. It should be made clear in the family that, as soon as he improves, he will again be expected to 'pull his weight.' This situation is identical to any other where a family member suffers an illness, say a broken leg, and needs time to recuperate.

The danger is that the schizophrenic may grow to prefer his 'preferential status' to what he sees as the burdens and complexities of being well. He may decide that improvement is not worth it. This is a possibility with all illnesses, including broken legs. Some relatives worry about this possibility too much, some not enough. This is an issue that is very important to discuss with the individual involved, his therapist, and other family members. If the patient becomes a 'tyrant' there is a need for counseling or family therapy.

Helping with sexual concerns

Although the expression of sexual urges may be disturbed in schizophrenia, sexual performance itself is intact, as are sexual feelings. Expression may be inhibited by fear, guilt, embarrassment, or lack of opportunity. Without means of expression, the person with schizophrenia may appear to lack sexual urges or he may express sexuality inappropriately. This can result from a lack of experience or from misinterpretation of other people's intent.

Lack of experience results from early onset of this illness, which often strikes in adolescence or early adulthood before dating and social skills are fully developed. After the acute illness, it is sometimes difficult to make up for the critical time lost. A person's confidence may be shattered and he may feel unattractive and undesirable.

This lack of confidence is hard to overcome, which is perhaps the reason why the majority of people with schizophrenia never marry. This is truer for men than for women, since the man traditionally is expected to take charge in dating and courting. Especially for those who do not marry, shyness and lack of opportunity make sexual relationships difficult, although social skills training, social clubs, and sex education help to overcome this difficulty.

Misinterpretation of other people's intent may occur when, for instance, a person thinks that certain hand gestures imply that the other person is sexually interested. Convinced of this mistaken belief, the male patient may openly proposition a woman whom he hardly knows. Not infrequently a patient may mistakenly believe that others think that he is homosexual. In his mind he must prove to them they are wrong so, again, he may press his suit inappropriately on a woman with whom he is barely acquainted.

Sometimes sexual thoughts, which are of course universal but which most people keep to themselves, come to the surface and are blurted out. It may happen that people with a schizophrenic illness interpose into everyday conversations comments such as: 'Is it okay to play with yourself? Are you looking at my genitals? How many times a week do you have sex?' These are disconcerting to the unprepared listener but they are not dangerous in the sense that the person thus preoccupied is about to act on uninhibited sexual impulses. These questions are best answered matter-of-factly without undue emotional reactions.

Some persons with schizophrenia seem to flee actively from interpersonal sexuality. They become very anxious at the thought of sex and learn to satisfy their sexual urges through fantasy and masturbation. Masturbation should not be a cause for concern unless it is truly excessive or occurs in socially unacceptable situations. On occasion it makes the individual feel unduly guilty and this requires reassurance. There are, of course, individual variations in sex drive and these issues require nonjudgmental airing and discussion. If sexual preoccupations are not allayed by reassurance and discussion. and if they appear to take on delusional proportions, it is wisest to suggest that the patient bring the matter up with his doctor or therapist.

Sex therapy techniques that are behavioral and aimed at reducing anxiety and increasing confidence may also be helpful to the schizophrenic patient with sexual problems. These are most effective when the patient is in a relationship and when both partners can attend sessions. The patient's therapist may be able to conduct these sessions, or he may refer the patient elsewhere for this more specific kind of counseling.

The drugs that are used in schizophrenia (the neuroleptics) have direct and indirect effects on hormones and on other chemical transmitters which control sexual functioning. The antidepressants and the antiparkinsonians may also have effects which interfere with erection and ejaculation in males. These side-effects may be temporary until the dose is correctly adjusted but, nevertheless, they may have profound psychological impact on the affected person. In women, antipsychotic medication may disrupt menstruation and may decrease sexual interest and interfere with orgasm. It is difficult to know if the latter occurs frequently because women rarely complain of it. It may be that this is a private worry which is not easily brought to the medical person's attention. Often patients attribute the sexual changes to other things and do not think of the medication as a possible cause. Families need to be aware of this and to encourage patients to discuss these issues openly. It may not be difficult to solve this problem with appropriate changes of drug or dosage.

There is, of course, much more to sexual concerns than the mechanics of sex. Intimacy is a difficult area for those who have been schizophrenic, as is commitment and the sustaining of relationships. Families need to be available to discuss the responsibilities involved, to cushion the hurts, to encourage some experimentation, and to advise on matters of contraception, sexually transmitted diseases, and sexual counseling. Interference with menstruation is a very common side-effect of drugs. Many women on neuroleptics do not menstruate and, on this issue, families can be reassuring. It does not, of course, mean that the nonmenstruating woman is invulnerable to pregnancy. Precautions against both unwanted pregnancy and disease need to be taken. This is important especially for schizophrenic women who may be overcompliant to the demands of others or, alternatively, rebellious against societal rules. In other words, they may be at special risk.

Helping a depressed patient

Symptoms of depression should never be taken lightly and are best reported to the doctor or therapist. Depression means feeling helpless and hopeless. Guilt and self-recrimination are usually part of it. So are listlessness, insomnia, lack of appetite, and lack of desire to do anything at all. Often it is accompanied by thoughts of suicide.

There is no magic answer to depression. Try to stand by and be patient. Do not blame a person for being depressed. He cannot help it. He may not be able to talk or to say what is on his mind. Do not expect him to. Be prepared to sit with him in silence. Try and say things and do things that will make him feel better about himself. Encourage exercise, good food, good sleeping habits, and socializing, but do not let yourself get frustrated if he balks at your suggestions. Do not let yourself get depressed, too. Depressed people are very draining. You will need time away from each other. Depressions, fortunately, are self-limiting. They do not last forever. Psychotherapy, antidepressant medication, or ECT may help. In some schizo-affective patients a reduction in the dose of neuroleptic may be useful.

Helping an angry patient

Most of the time anger is related to depression, unhappiness, and fear. Try to calm your relative's fears. Anger is often provoked by uncertainties or inconsistencies. Try to be clear and predictable. Try not to react angrily too readily.

Anger is a universal feeling, and, consequently, aggressive acts are common in all kinds of situations. Infants are born with a capacity for great rage and indeed the control of anger is part of the socialization that we all go through. We all have internal conflicts or external situations that lead us to angry feelings and often to fantasies of aggressive behavior.

Schizophrenia may have some significant impact on the occurrence of aggression within the family. There are some schizophrenics who become uninhibited when they are acutely psychotic. Occasionally mothers with schizophrenia may become uninhibited and may abuse or neglect their children. During the illness some patients form a delusion of a paranoid nature involving ideas of revenge against others or the fantasy of needing to defend themselves against imminent attack. Sometimes patients may have auditory hallucinations that command them to violent acts. Of a similar nature are repeated thoughts having to do with aggression, though these rarely lead to action.

Generally angry outbursts are reflections of the illness. The management is mainly medical. Comforting the patient with non-confronting remarks, food, or the opportunity of privacy may produce calmer attitudes. If necessary the police may have to be called to get the patient to a doctor, but once the patient is at the hospital it is the responsibility of the physician to treat the basic disorder that led to the violent behavior.

Perhaps more common is the problem of hostility within the family when the patient is already in the recovery phase. The individual may be very frustrated by his illness, which he perceives as delaying the development of his life. He may hold the relatives responsible. The parents or spouse or indeed other members of the family may feel guilty about the patient's illness and also resentful of the demands the sickness has placed upon them. At the same time, the patient is also feeling guilty and resentful. It is common to find in such situations mutual criticism and high levels of expressed emotion. This is an atmosphere in which aggression may arise and this may be not only from the patient towards the family members but from other family members towards the patient. If such episodes are recurrent, there is clearly a need for physical separation, time away from one another, and also for family counseling.

Helping with legal trouble

Sometimes poor judgment or psychotic thinking may lead to actions that produce a legal charge; most are laid under traffic laws. Practice varies from community to community, but the crown attorney (Canada) or district attorney (United States) may be prepared to drop the charge or diminish the penalty if he is contacted directly by the relatives, if the nature of the schizo-phrenic illness is explained, if he is assured that the patient is under psychiatric treatment and that the family is available and strongly supportive. An up-to-date psychiatric assessment including diagnosis, severity, type of treatment, and prognosis (outlook) should be made available to the defence lawyer if the case is prosecuted.

Coping with death

Death of a family member or a close friend is an inescapable reality and a person with schizophrenia must face it as everyone else must. It is a major stress, but the recovering schizophrenic cannot be shielded from it. It cannot be avoided or denied. If possible, the schizophrenic family member should be prepared for it by repeated family discussions.

The involvement of the schizophrenic individual in the events surrounding the death should be as full as possible. He has to be given a chance to say his last farewell like everyone else. At times of major family stress, such as illness and bereavement, the schizophrenic is often a tower of strength. It is as if reality, at those times, has finally impinged on his consciousness and has overpowered the mysterious and frightening fantasies that so frequently hold sway.

When the supporting relatives die

This is a concern relatives frequently mention. It is the best reason to encourage independent living for the ex-patient while the close family can still help. There are few schizophrenics who cannot learn to look after themselves or find their way about once their illness reaches a stable phase. Upon the death of the supporting relative there may be a brief relapse, with readmission to hospital if necessary. Subsequent support from other relatives will usually be all that is needed. When this is not possible, life in a supervised residence is the best alternative.

Is it better to live at home?

Families sometimes think it is better for their relative to be at home, but this may not be so. Individuals with schizophrenia usually do better in a home where there is not too much commotion and where the general level of expressed feelings is low. But arguments, disagreements, and quarrels are part of family life. Some families try to avoid quarrels, to pretend disagreements never occur – this is not a good idea because it makes things unclear to the schizo- phrenic. He finds it hard to understand what is going on. However, loud voices and shouting matches are frightening and may provoke a return of symptoms in the patient, especially if minor criticisms lead to overwhelming accusations. An example of this is a request to make the bed which leads on to more sweeping statements about the patient 'never caring for those who love him.' Sometimes life in a boarding home or a group home for ex-patients is more calm and involves less emotional pressure. In the long run this may be to the schizophrenic's benefit.

It may happen that an ex-patient cannot manage to live on his own but refuses to move away from home to a boarding house or supervised residence. And yet at home he may be quite difficult to live with. It is hard for families to ask a patient to leave, but having him at home may be disrupting to him and to the rest of the family. It is important to remember that a decision that the patient *not* live at home does not necessarily denote a lack of caring and is not an admission of failure. It may well be the wisest course of action. However, such important steps should always be taken in full consultation with the therapist so that appropriate back-up or 'rescue' plans can be instituted easily.

Case vignette
Patients with schizophrenia are said to change address often. This is true of one woman who spent January and February in hospital, March in her own one-room self-contained apartment, April and

May in a group home, June in the hospital, July and August in a flat with her boyfriend, September in her father's home, October in her sister's home, and November back with her boyfriend.

How much supervision?

The need for supervision varies. The extent of social recovery that the person has achieved and the amount of responsibility he can take on usually dictate the amount and the nature of supervision required. For example, a person who has made a full social recovery is essentially on his own. He will need to keep on with his treatment, but he will look after that himself and the family does not need constantly to check on him.

At certain stages of the illness, however, the family needs to make sure that the patient attends his treatment sessions, does not forget to take his medication, gets up on time in the morning to attend his classes, does not fight with others in the family, does not forget to shower and shave, and so on.

Unpredictable behavior and impulsive actions can occur in schizophrenia. For instance, the schizophrenic may suddenly decide to leave home or quit work, or to get drunk or smoke pot, to yell at a neighbor or to invite strangers into the house, or to engage in irresponsible sexual behavior or attempt suicide. These are not everyday occurrences but they may happen, especially during periods of turmoil. It is not realistic to expect a parent or friend to anticipate and prevent all such occurrences. If something untoward does happen, do not jump to the conclusion that you are to blame, that closer supervision might have prevented it. Often individuals, including schizophrenics, learn only from their mistakes. Learning from experience is an important part of becoming self-sufficient. Speak to the individual and his therapist about the amount of supervision that is required at various stages of illness.

What is 'overinvolvement'?

When a schizophrenic patient is ill, he may be unable to participate in discussions between his therapist and his family. At these times it may occasionally be simpler for the therapist to talk with relatives alone. When the patient has recovered enough to take part in the talks, most doctors or therapists prefer that he be present. Ideally there should be nothing that needs to be said to the therapist that cannot be said in the patient's presence. For the family to confide in the therapist in private, with the request that the conversation be kept secret, puts the therapist into a very uncomfortable position. Therapists will listen if one has something urgent to say, but will tell the patient what was said. This is part of the patient-therapist understanding.

The therapist-patient relationship and its confidentiality is important. Strictly speaking, the therapist cannot talk to relatives about intimate details of the illness and treatment without the patient's permission. This is difficult for relatives to understand, especially when they feel they have something urgent to communicate. If a therapist, for whatever reason, ever refuses to answer a telephone call, write him a note that lists all the important facts he needs to know. Tell the patient you have done so.

Support of interested relatives is very valuable for the schizophrenic. He may, however, not always accept this. He may interpret interest and support as intrusiveness and 'meddling.' In that case it is better to back off and stand by in case of need, rather than to actively involve yourself. Ask your relative's therapist for guidance in this, as it is an important issue.

Case vignette
One patient's mother phoned his doctor after each appointment to ask if he had gotten there and to ask what he had said. The patient reported that she listened in while he spoke on the phone and made sure he took his medications by dissolving them in his tea. The mother meant well but was overinvolved.

Money

Most schizophrenics are able to maintain control of their own finances. During difficult periods there may be times when someone other than the patient should be looking after his financial affairs. If he is squandering his assets unwisely because of illness, the physician can make out a certificate of financial incompetence. This does not commit the patient to hospital, but legally turns his financial affairs over to another party, a private or a public trustee. This kind of overseeing of the patient's financial affairs may be necessary for short or sometimes for longer periods.

Making a will

Relatives should consult with the family lawyer about providing for the patient after they die. Large inheritances can be placed in investment securities and a monthly trust fund can be established for a disabled relative. It is wise to think ahead and reassuring to know that a family member with a disability will be well looked after, no matter what happens.

Is schizophrenia a reason for divorce?

If the illness exists prior to marriage, the spouse knew what to expect and is usually more tolerant and accepting. If the illness arises after marriage, it is often very difficult for the spouse. Frequently the schizophrenic and his family blame the spouse, and the spouse ends up blaming herself without cause. When there are small children in the family, this may provide extra strain and burden. A person suffering from schizophrenia may be unable to fulfill a parental role and the spouse may feel like a single parent, a wage earner, and a nurse, all rolled into one. This may cause great resentment and may end in divorce. All love relationships are hard at times and there is no question that schizophrenia can place heavy burdens on marriages.

If the question of separation or divorce comes up, try to be clear about what is making the situation intolerable. If it is illness-related behavior on the part of the schizophrenic, can that be eliminated by proper treatment? Will it be better in time? Try to sort this out with your spouse and his therapist. Is the problem a financial one? Is the individual's ability to earn a good living the problem? Is the problem his difficulty in being a parent, a lover, or an emotional support to you? How much of the problem has to do with your spouse's personality, quite apart from his illness? How much of the problem is the interaction between the two of you, again separate from schizophrenia? These are difficult questions to untangle. They will require discussions with your spouse, his family and friends, your family and friends, the therapist, a lawyer, and possibly a religious counselor. Try to talk with people who understand schizophrenia.

Can schizophrenics help relatives?

When an individual has recognized that he has a serious illness and that it is his responsibility to look after himself, the relatives' lot becomes much easier. Acceptance of illness is not easy and usually takes time. Once it has come about, the relatives can relax. Once the ex-patient has taken on the task of looking after his own well-being, he will make it his business to learn as much as possible about all aspects of schizophrenia and will comply more or less enthusiastically with the treatment plan. At this point he now becomes a resource person for the relatives. The schizophrenic needs to ask questions about his disease, to report all symptoms, to talk freely to his therapist about his worries and concerns, to be aware of the effects of his medication, and to take pride in his strengths and accomplishments. Once he has taken on the full responsibility of maintaining his own health, the relatives become less tense and worried and, in turn, become easier to live with and enjoy.

How should relatives and friends respond?

People usually want to be as helpful as they can be to those in distress, and so they look for the best ways to respond to a schizophrenic relative or friend. Perhaps it would be helpful to know that there is no best way, and that sadness, anger, shame, and avoidance are natural ways in which individuals often respond to life crises.

This is true no matter what the crisis is. It is natural at first to ignore the problem, hoping it will go away. If it nevertheless persists, most people look for someone to blame. Pinning blame on ourselves or others, on God or on the government, on the doctors or nurses, seems to lessen the torment.

Nobody wants to blame the victim, in this case the patient. Sparing him, however, can lead to suppressed rage and disappointment towards him and perhaps to unrealistic blame and undeserved anger directed towards others. While the patient is, of course, not responsible for the onset of his illness, he must, along with many others, take responsibility for his treatment and, ultimately, for his improvement.

Families and friends usually find that after the first shock and adaptation they begin to share the responsibility and begin to delegate the many tasks at hand. Some are tasks for the patient, some for the doctors and agencies, some for relatives. Some tasks are accomplished well, but others fail, which may lead to a fresh cycle of frustration and disappointment.

None of this response, of course, is specific to schizophrenia. Life crises of all kinds lead to chaotic emotions, but they are also times of opportunity. It is important to realize that stress and unhappiness are to be expected, and that most relatives will be able to cope without professional help. Many, however, find it helpful to share their feelings with someone who understands – for example, others in similar situations. If the emotional responses are difficult to bear, many find it useful to seek help from a psychotherapist. The better the relative can come to terms with his own emotions, the more help he can be to the patient.

SIX

Outcome

When a person is ill, he wants to know when he will feel better. He wants to know how long the most troublesome symptoms will last. He wants to know whether, at the end of the illness, he will be feeling his usual self. He wants to know whether there is any risk that he will feel worse, rather than better, over time. Can this illness prove fatal? Are there people who never recover? Will it ever come back, and if it does, will it be milder or more severe than the first time? What effect will this illness have on career, marriage, and general health? What preparations, accommodations, acceptances have to be made? What can be done to speed recovery, prevent recurrence, enhance treatment, and improve the quality of life if the illness lingers?

Although there is much that we do not know about schizophrenia, some of these questions can be answered.

How soon will I feel better?

The answer to this is that it varies. Most typically, acute schizophrenia is self-limited to several months after which most of the symptoms wane. This, of course, depends on appropriate treatment. After the acute period is over, however, the patient may not immediately feel better. He will regret the time lost, be mystified and frightened by what has happened, and worried about the future. He will be not quite himself because of drug side-effects and because the acute illness has sapped him of energy and ambition. Although the most troubling symptoms will have disappeared, he will not feel his usual self. Some people go through a period of actually feeling worse, more depressed about what happened, and less optimistic about the future. In retrospect the actual illness may not feel so bad, and there is a tendency to blame the treatment rather than the illness for some of the associated problems. There is usually a convalescent period of some months, after which the patient starts getting back to the business of living.

Can this illness prove fatal?

One does not die of schizophrenia but schizophrenia can lead to death by suicide or by neglect of hygiene and health and safety. The death rate is higher for these reasons among schizophrenics than among the population at large.

Are there people who never recover?

Most patients worry that they'll be 'locked up forever.' This is a historical holdover from times when severe mental illness led to indefinite, sometimes permanent, hospitalization. This no longer happens. There are people with very severe forms who, for many years, seem not to recover. In general, the first 5 to 10 years are the most severe for these people. After that, improvement does take place, even among the most ill. For those whose illness seems to be taking this severe, chronic, unremitting course, it is important to remember that there is a light at the end of the tunnel. Schizophrenia weakens its hold in the 40s and usually by the 60s formerly very ill people feel quite good. This may seem like too long to wait but, in contrast with most other illnesses, it is actually optimistic. Most illnesses get worse with time and more and more debilitating. This is not the case with schizophrenia.

Will the illness come back?

Typically schizophrenia comes and goes. In some people the recurrences are few and far between; in others they come so frequently that they seem to blend into each other. The frequency, again, diminishes with age. Recurrences are sometimes more severe than early attacks, but sometimes less so. There is no general rule about this that holds true for everyone, except that the first ten years are usually worse than whatever follows later.

What is the effect on career, marriage, quality of life?

Schizophrenia has a profound effect on life plans. As is discussed in various parts of the book, this illness interferes with friendships, intimacy, family relationships, schooling, work, enjoyment, activity, ambition, and self-esteem. The person with schizophrenia must deal with a much harsher reality than others need to and must adapt to and conquer far greater odds. He needs all the strength, support, education, sympathy, and guidance possible. He cannot do it on his own completely. Family and friends must assist, although the person with schizophrenia must also gradually learn to take responsibility for his illness and for enriching his own life in the fullest possible way.

What can be done?

There are numerous avenues of help which are described in this book. The worst possibility is to feel helpless and to think that nothing one does matters. This is not true in schizophrenia. There are many directions for the patient and the family to take which will make the burden of illness lighter and which will speed recovery.

Antipsychotic drugs block the symptoms of acute illness and are a great advance in treatment. They are only a partial answer because they do not reverse all symptoms and induce side-effects of their own. Understanding, morale-boosting, rehabilitation techniques, and family education methods help in many ways. Research continues and new understanding will produce better treatments and improve outcome. Until then there is comfort in knowing that schizophrenic episodes become rarer and less severe with age, and the psychosocial deficiencies, so apparent in young adulthood, wane considerably as the person matures.

SEVEN

Support for relatives

Introduction

Schizophrenic illness presents family and friends with many crises. As with all crises, there are many individuals and agencies who would want to help. At times they do not know how to. Sometimes they try but give the wrong advice. Knowing the right person to turn to in a crisis is very important.

Help in case of 'relapse'

When symptoms have more or less disappeared, one speaks of *remission*. When symptoms reappear to a significant degree, one talks of *relapse*. Relapses are distressing for schizophrenics and relatives, though somewhat less so when anticipated and planned for. Schizophrenia, for the most part, is a 'relapsing' condition, so it makes sense to expect return of symptoms and not to be caught off guard.

It is best not to wait until the symptoms become severe but to act early. The time to be worried is when the person first starts behaving in the way he did prior to his first illness. It is safe to assume that similar behavior means similar preoccupations on his mind. The first step is to ask the person what is worrying him.

The next step is to suggest that the psychiatrist or the therapist be informed. If the person is reluctant to do so and you care for him, then tell him of your concern and that you are going to contact his therapist.

If the therapist is unavailable, the best person to contact is the family doctor. In some communities, in an emergency, he can make a home visit. He may be able to evaluate the situation over the phone and make further recommendations, or he may contact the hospital. A public health nurse or, in some communities, a mental health nurse will also make a home visit. The earlier the situation is attended to the more likely will be the ill person's willingness to co-operate. Most hospital emergency departments are open 24 hours a day, seven days a week.

What to do if the individual refuses help

Try to find out why he is refusing. He may have a logical or an illogical reason. Sometimes he is afraid he will be hospitalized, or given a particular form of treatment he dislikes, or will be attended by a particular person he dislikes. Sometimes it is possible to assure him that this will not be the case.

Often the individual has, by wishful thinking, convinced himself that he would never have a return of symptoms. Perhaps the family also, by wishful thinking, has encouraged him to believe this. So when symptoms do return, it is tempting to deny them. Being prepared for the worst makes the worst not so bad. After an episode of schizophrenic illness, there is a 70 percent risk of having a second episode within the year if the patient is not on medication. If the patient *is* on medication, this risk is reduced to 30 percent. With very careful follow-up and intervention (temporarily raising the dose of medication or stepping up the frequency of appointments) subsequent hospitalizations can often be avoided. It is best to talk to your relative from time to time about the possibility of relapse and to plan together what should be done if that happens.

Often when the patient is adamantly refusing to see his therapist or denying that there is anything amiss, there may be one or two other people who can get through to him. Among these one should consider other relatives, friends, employer or colleagues, minister, or, occasionally, fellow patients.

Who can help?

Serious disturbance
If the patient is obviously very disturbed but continues absolutely to refuse psychiatric help, the family members will have to acquaint themselves with the mental health laws in their community to see what can be done. Certain measures can be taken.

Either the family physician or the treating psychiatrist comes to the house and, if necessary, can legally certify the patient as being mentally ill and in need of hospitalization. In some communities the patient must be brought by the relatives to the evaluation service. Generally involuntary hospitalization can only take place if, in addition to illness, there is the likelihood that the patient will be harmful to himself or to others, or if he is in great danger, for example, from hunger, untreated physical illness, or other self-neglect.

If the patient is threatening to harm himself or other people, the police have to be called. Forewarn the police about the person's likely behavior and the reasons for it. Some communities have 'community officers' who are not in uniform. This may be less frightening to the patient and less upsetting to the family. Many specially trained officers, though not all, are very humane in their dealings with the mentally ill.

Because of unfamiliarity with their responsibility and liability in these circumstances, doctors or police may respond only in a limited way. This may be especially true in communities where mental health laws have undergone changes and nobody knows for sure what the new regulations are. The local psychiatric hospital or department of health information service can be contacted for information on the law and on appropriate procedures for ensuring the patient's safe conduct to a hospital. In some areas the public health department will send a nurse to evaluate the situation. She may be able to persuade the patient to take medication on a doctor's order. Most mental health laws do not permit treating the patient, that is, giving medication, against his will, except under special circumstances. The nurse would know which doctor or which police officer to call to fill out the legal forms and escort the patient to hospital.

In communities where doctors are scarce or where the doctor cannot examine the patient, relatives may be allowed to give evidence under oath in front of a justice of the peace or magistrate to the effect that the patient is seriously ill and potentially dangerous to himself or to others. An order may then be issued to the police for the patient to be taken to the nearest hospital for an assessment.

Some hospital psychiatric departments have special teams that will come to the house in an emergency. They will assess the patient and suggest a treatment plan. In some cases they will arrange for immediate hospitalization, even against the patient's will, if they see evidence of serious mental illness and potential harm. Mental health legislation varies from country to country, state to state, and province to province. It always favors informal or voluntary hospitalization, reserving involuntary hospitalization for those who are ill and at danger and unwilling to seek treatment.

Most mental health laws authorize the police to bring individuals to hospital for psychiatric assessment of several days' duration if they witness bizarre or dangerous behavior, if they have a doctor's certificate to that effect or a judicial warrant. At the end of the assessment period, if there is sufficient cause, the individual may be kept in hospital for a further period, against his will if necessary.

Some families convince their ill relative by weight of numbers. In a demonstration of solidarity and strength, many family members together are able to obtain the patient's co-operation in going for treatment. Crises sometimes have this paradoxical capacity to bring the family unit closer and unite it in a common purpose.

Violence
Threats of violence and actual violence, including verbal abuse and attacks on property and persons, can occur when schizophrenics are agitated, deluded, and frightened. These can make the home atmosphere intolerable. A threatening approach to the patient is not helpful. Try to remain calm and avoid arguments and counterattacks. An overstimulating environment makes things worse. Try to reassure him of his safety and that help is available. Families are sometimes embarrassed to involve others, but the presence of nonthreatening friends or neighbors can defuse a difficult situation. Other people need simply to be there; they do not need to interact or involve themselves with the patient. Make sure that the patient also has the opportunity for privacy, which may be essential for him. Do not hesitate to call for police assistance and state your case as strongly as possible.

Withdrawal
It is common for schizophrenics to become increasingly and painfully shy and withdrawn. This can be very frustrating to relatives who would sometimes rather provoke a spark of anger than be faced day-in and day-out with a wall of seeming indifference. It can be embarrassing in front of others to have your family member hide in his room, or avoid looking people in the eye, or insist that you stay home with him. It is important to remember that such embarrassment is not necessarily a reason to spoil your own life and your relative's too. Friends and neighbors need not be avoided. The better they know the patient, the more comfortable they will be with him and he with them. Your life must go on and the schizophrenic family member will gradually adapt to your routines, schedules, social life, and work life. In the long run you are helping him to overcome his withdrawal by not capitulating to his demands for your constant protection. It is essential for your sake, and ultimately for his, that you live as full a life as possible.

Talk of suicide

Some schizophrenic patients can become quite depressed. These mood changes often reflect an understandable reaction to the illness. Vulnerable people may fear relapse and failure. They may blame themselves for their illness. The rate of suicide reported in most clinics for schizophrenia is considerably higher than that for the general population. Suicide usually does not occur at the very beginning of illness, when the individual involved does not really believe he is ill. And it does not usually come when he has come to terms with his illness. It is more frequent in the in-between stage, when the realization is new and not yet accepted.

Talk of suicide, no matter how vague, should be reported immediately. The reference to death is not always direct, but may consist of pessimistic or sad statements, such as 'What's the point?' Phone the hospital emergency at any hour. Ensure that the patient's therapist be informed and that he see the patient as soon as possible. Frequent personal contacts with the therapist are helpful. Hospitalization may or may not be necessary. Antidepressants or ECT may be prescribed or neuroleptic medications altered. Encouragement from relatives and friends often helps the patient to feel less of a disappointment and a burden to everyone.

If the patient does attempt suicide, relatives must try not to blame themselves. The person with schizophrenia is prone to many imaginings, with sudden changes not uncommon. He may misread and misinterpret events around him and experience acute depression. Knowing that this can happen takes away some of the anguish and self-blame. When a tragedy happens, it is human nature to look for someone to shoulder the blame: oneself, the doctor or therapist, friends. The apportioning of blame helps one to survive the pain and loss. The real blame lies with the nature of the disease.

The treatment team

It is important to maintain regular contact with the treatment team. In most cases relatives will be interviewed by a member of the team, often by a social worker. The family's collaboration in providing additional information is essential for diagnosis, treatment, and planning for discharge. Some hospitalized patients might insist that their relatives not be contacted. This can place the treatment team in a quandary because the patient's wishes have to be respected. In most instances, however, the family is kept informed and consulted prior to discharge. If you find that you are not contacted, take the initiative yourself. The family may *provide* information with no rupture of the patient's right to confidentiality.

It is your responsibility when speaking to the treatment team to ask direct questions. Do not hesitate to question the diagnosis, the treatment, the outlook, and so on. Do not hesitate to ask for a second opinion if you have any doubts. Try not to be discouraged by what is almost inescapable hospital routine: waiting, postponement, changing shifts, staff turnover, one person sometimes contradicting what another has said. This should not happen but often does. Most hospital personnel are well-intentioned but are often very busy and not always up-to-date on the latest team decisions. Do not be upset if you are asked not to visit for a period when your relative is very disturbed, but do keep in touch with the team.

Community resources

Schizophrenic patients are often involved with many helping agencies. These are described from the patient's point of view in Chapter 3. Also see Appendixes I and II. Many of the same agencies have staff that, because they know the patient, can also be helpful to relatives. The community offers a variety of rehabilitation programs such as day treatment centers, vocational services, volunteer services, and self-help groups. In addition there are mental health agencies, public health nurses, community occupational therapists, and social workers. There are also family practitioners, general physicians, and psychiatrists. Do not hesitate to contact the local mental health division in your area for information.

Will there be more support for relatives?

Understanding and support for the families of schizophrenics will certainly increase in the coming years. The burden and responsibility of families have become clearer to mental health professionals over the last 15 years.

Self-help programs initiated by relatives all over the world have been growing in popularity and have already produced extensive recommendations for improved health care (see Appendix II). As time goes on, there will be more emphasis on family strength – those forces that contribute to a more solid family unit and those factors that foster and develop coping mechanisms in each family member. There will also be increased efforts to educate the public about schizophrenia. There exists strong research evidence that relatives are not to blame. This information needs to be disseminated to the public at large.

One outcome of self-help programs will be the accumulated experience of relatives about what does and what does not work in the everyday interaction with schizophrenic relatives. There will be efforts to pool this large natural resource – the relatives – into an effective and politically powerful organization.

National organizations, such as the National Alliance for the Mentally Ill, the National Schizophrenia Fellowship in the United Kingdom, and the Canadian Friends of Schizophrenics, will grow. They are essential in helping to reduce the family's burden and in pointing out current gaps in the provision of mental health services.

EIGHT

Work and school

Back to school and work

A minority of schizophrenic patients show a complete return to their previous functioning when stabilized on neuroleptics. Most, however, show some disability, sometimes because of mild residual symptoms and often because of psychological reactions to the illness.

It is nevertheless quite feasible to return to school or work after an episode of schizophrenia, although there is usually a period during which attention and concentration are not nearly at the same level as they were prior to onset of the illness.

Often ex-patients are ambivalent about returning to the workforce or have misgivings about returning to school after having lost a number of months of schooling. They often lack confidence in their ability to cope with their classes or jobs. It helps if the doctor, with the patient's permission, has kept the employer or teacher informed of the patient's progress. Vocational or scholastic assessments are useful to restore self-confidence. Some mental health centers have a teacher or vocational counselor on staff who may act as a consultant. It may be possible for the patient to train for work even before discharge from hospital. A temporary period in a sheltered and supervised setting may be beneficial.

Once working or in school, an employee or student is either competent or not. Medical diagnoses should not be an issue except when it comes to time off for medical treatment. Some employers and teachers, however, worry about someone with a diagnosis of schizophrenia. Much of the worry stems from not knowing what the term implies. We hope that this book will dispel some of the mystery. Problems will become less of a hindrance if an employer or teacher and the therapist can discuss them. Not all of the school- or work-related problems are found in every patient. As with other people, the start of a new job or class is often the critical point. Employers and teachers can help by structuring the situation early on.

Punctuality

Many individuals with a history of schizophrenia find it difficult to get up in the morning and face the day. Time pressures, crowded buses, snarled traffic – universal problems – loom large. The result is that being late for work in the morning is not infrequent. Employees with a history of schizophrenia do best in jobs where the hours are flexible. They often prefer shift work, especially working those shifts when they are relatively alone.

Passivity

Employers and teachers sometimes complain that the person with schizophrenia shows relatively little initiative, takes instructions passively, or shows little enthusiasm for the job. Some of the seeming passivity covers up anxiety and discomfort. When the person feels more comfortable, the real interest will start to show through. At any rate, not all jobs or studies require enthusiasm. Industry and reliability are usually more important.

Time off

For some schizophrenics long-term commitments are frightening.

There may be a strong temptation to leave a new job or class and never come back because of the fear and, sometimes, the conviction that no one will notice anyway, that no one will care. This is a real problem for many people with schizophrenia, and many potentially good jobs get sabotaged in this way. The understanding employer or teacher should telephone a person who misses work and express interest and concern. Once he knows he is missed and that his work really counts for something, the problem may be over.

Stress

The schizophrenic person does not handle stress particularly well. Highly stressed work with many deadlines and constant evaluation and competition is probably not the right kind. Schizophrenics tend to see people as more stress-inducing than machines. The fewer people around, the better.

Clear instructions

People with schizophrenia are not good at reading between the lines. They tend to read *too much* between the lines and assume, when the message is not clear, that they are being criticized or put down. The message has to be very clear. Work instructions have to be simple and precise. One instruction at a time is easier to cope with than many given at once. Once a routine is established, everything becomes much easier.

Anger

People with schizophrenia get angry no more frequently or forcibly than anyone else. The only difference is that their anger is often unexpected and seemingly unprovoked. Because it seems to come out of nowhere, it is often difficult to cope with. Usually it is caused by reading something into what someone has said or misinterpreting something someone has done. It can be avoided or quickly quelled if the person explains what it is that was said or done and what was intended.

Moodiness

If a schizophrenic's moods seem very changeable and there is much irritability, it may be a sign of the return of active symptoms. It helps if the employer or teacher has the kind of relationship with the employee or student where this type of problem can be openly discussed and a recommendation to get in touch with the therapist can be made. Frankness is preferable to complaints about the employee to others.

Slowness

Teachers or employers may notice slowness on the part of schizophrenic students or employees and wonder if this is caused by the medication used to treat schizophrenia. In some instances the slowness may be due to medication; in other instances it may be a result of preoccupation. If the job requires speedy work and the person is incapable of it, it may be best to suggest a different job rather than to demand the impossible.

Isolation

A preference for being alone should not unduly worry the employer or teacher. Often the schizophrenic person does better work when he is by himself and away from interpersonal stress.

Preoccupation

Preoccupation may be a sign of worry about doing the job well. It may, however, signal problems. If this worries the employer or teacher, he should feel free to approach the employee or student and ask him about it.

Appointments with a therapist

It is important that the student or employee be able to continue his regular appointments for medication and counseling. Some doctors and clinics have evening hours, but many do not. Allowing regular time for appointments, even if it means missing time from work or school, safeguards the employee's or the student's health and his work.

It is often helpful if the employer or teacher, with the schizophrenic's consent, has an opportunity to talk to the therapist. In some instances, particularly early on in the employment or school year, it might be possible to arrange for an on-the-spot visit by the therapist.

Special settings

Many schizophrenics are never able to enter the competitive workforce, and for these people there exist in most communities sheltered work settings and special vocational placements. These may be required temporarily, for a training and adjustment period, or for prolonged periods. Pay is a problem since a person working a full day deserves at least a minimum wage, and special programs are unable to provide this.

Conclusion

Those persons with a history of schizophrenia who *are* able to work competitively usually become loyal, reliable, and valued employees.

Case vignette
One 48-year-old patient has held the same job for 20 years and has never missed a day's work with the exception of three short sick leaves during which she was hospitalized for severe paranoid symptoms. Otherwise, although probably always hearing voices and attributing them to persecution by her first psychiatrist, she has maintained steady employment and is considered very good at her work.

NINE

The future

Changing public attitudes

Attitudes towards schizophrenia have changed to a considerable degree. Since the 1950s, particularly since the introduction of effective pharmacological treatment in 1952, more and more schizophrenics live in the community rather than in psychiatric hospitals. This has allowed the public to come into contact with recovered patients. More and more people have come to realize that there is no reason to be frightened of schizophrenia. Not everyone, however, has been fortunate enough to have had first-hand contact with recovered patients. Many people still live in fear of schizophrenia, imagining the sufferer to possess two unpredictable personalities, a Dr Jekyll and a Mr Hyde.

Such a view cannot persist much longer, because it is so far from the truth. There has been continuing education about schizophrenia, and the more this continues the faster public attitudes will change. The stigma attached to mental illness as a whole, though still present, is not as pronounced as it once was. More and more relatives and ex-patients are speaking openly about schizophrenia. They will, undoubtedly, become a powerful force in changing public opinion.

More facilities

Hospitals, rehabilitation centers, and community support systems already exist. Some areas have more facilities than others, usually because a local pressure group of interested persons was able to stimulate interest, change local bylaws, and garner funds. Interested, knowledgeable, and highly motivated groups of people are the keys to improving present supports and developing new ones. For example, in most communities there continues to be an unmet need for supervised group homes or apartments for those schizophrenics who have no family or who cannot live with their family. An organized group of interested nonprofessionals working together could do much towards developing such facilities. The same applies to the need for social and vocational programs.

As new, still experimental programs for rehabilitation prove successful, there will be a need to expand them so that all schizophrenic patients can reap the same benefits. Staying abreast of new developments in the treatment of schizophrenia and working together politically to make sure that successful treatment strategies are implemented in local communities are challenging and eminently worthwhile tasks for relatives. (See Appendix II for existing relatives' groups.) Pressure on government must emphasize the need for equitable funding for community-based programs.

Will there be a cure?

Cure means complete eradication of problems with no need for further treatment. There is no cure for schizophrenia. There is no cure at present for most medical disorders. Practically all illnesses, other than short-term infections, require continuous monitoring to ensure that symptoms do not reappear. So it is for schizophrenia. In the future, when the exact cause of illnesses, including schizophrenia, is better understood, the chances of finding a permanent cure will improve.

When most people ask about cure, however, they are thinking about control. They want to know, 'Will the patient get over his present problems and will he be able to resume his place in society?' The answer to this question, in most cases, is yes, although perhaps a qualified yes.

Forty years ago schizophrenic symptoms were so difficult to manage that two-thirds of individuals admitted to hospital for schizophrenia stayed there upwards of two years. Ten years ago, after effective drugs had been around for 20 years, only 1 in 10 patients needed a hospitalization of two years' duration. Today it is rare for patients to stay in hospital longer than 90 days. That is because of more effective medications and more widespread community supports for the convalescing patient.

If one looks at other indications of improvement (freedom from symptoms, employment record, interpersonal involvement, personal satisfaction, family's satisfaction) 80 percent of people with schizophrenia do well. With more research and better treatment, that percentage will increase and the extent of improvement will broaden.

Current research

Research into schizophrenia is burgeoning. Perhaps the fastest moving field of research right now is molecular genetics. New genetic techniques can help to locate the genes responsible for this illness and then, possibly, the gene products can be isolated and the basic cause of schizophrenia found. At the moment this possibility seems far off indeed, but considerable effort is going into investigating blood samples from families in which schizophrenia appears to run in order to try to find the gene(s) responsible.

Since schizophrenia appears to be caused not only by genes but also by environment, there is also considerable work going on in investigating the environment of the brain from conception on. This includes the study of the possible effects of trauma, infection, chemicals, and hormones, as well as psychological and social stressors.

New imaging techniques now allow us to look inside the brain while it works. In other words, a person's brain can be visualized while hallucinating or while attempting intellectual tasks. This may help us pinpoint which specific part of the brain malfunctions in schizophrenia.

Brain neurochemicals and hormones attach to specific receptor sides in the brain before triggering cellular communication. These receptors can also be visualized with the new imaging techniques, and this may help determine which receptors are defective or excessive.

Post-mortem study of persons with schizophrenia who have died also yields important information when such brains are carefully compared to others where schizophrenia was not present during life.

Psychological study of persons with schizophrenia is becoming more sophisticated as diagnosis is standardized and as psychophysiological test techniques improve. For instance, eye tracking is an interesting area of study. Schizophrenics, as well as close members of their families, frequently follow an object with their eyes in a manner which distinguishes them from nonschizophrenics. This may mean that the part of the brain that controls that particular eye motion is somehow affected in schizophrenia.

Another interesting finding is that schizophrenia, in contrast to most other diseases, seems to get better in old age. Since we know that nerve cells die as we get older, does this mean that the disease improves because defective cells die?

Also intriguing is the fact that schizophrenia is milder in women than in men. Do female hormones play a part?

There continues to be much we don't know. Why is the outlook for schizophrenia better in underdeveloped countries? Why do some people get completely better while others stay severely ill? Why do some respond well to available treatments and others not at all? Why are identical twins not always concordant for schizophrenia except when they are also identical for handedness? Why are more schizophrenics born in winter and early spring than at any other time? Why do some persons with schizophrenia suffer symptoms from childhood and others not become ill until middle age? Why do all effective antipsychotics currently available block receptors for dopamine and yet no dopamine excess has been demonstrated in schizophrenia? Why do symptoms in schizophrenia change over time? Why do some people with schizophrenia come from families where there is no schizophrenia but where there is a lot of depression or mania? What is the connection between marijuana or alcohol consumption or head trauma and the onset of schizophrenia? What are the effects of life experiences?

There are many unanswered questions about schizophrenia, and current research is attempting to try to answer them. Patients and families can help by volunteering to share their own experiences and by taking active part in research. They can also campaign for better research funding and, most of all, they can keep abreast of new developments. Popular science magazines usually report on new discoveries with enough detail to make them understandable.

PART TWO
Personal accounts

TEN

A mother's account

About five years ago, at the age of 24, our daughter became very disturbed: she was hearing voices, felt she was being followed, and her days and nights were filled with constant fear and anguish. Her father and I were puzzled and distraught. A few months later Elizabeth was admitted to hospital.

Though her father and I visited her each day of her four-month stay, we remained perplexed by her illness. During the entire period we never met her doctor. *We* had not asked for an appointment with him, and *he* had not requested to see us. Just prior to her discharge, we had an interview with the social worker, who briefly outlined some useful tips to help Elizabeth get established back home with us. She warned us to watch for certain danger signs that would indicate recurring illness. Plans would be made for Elizabeth to attend a sheltered workshop, and she would visit her own doctor on a regular basis to have her medication supervised.

The interview appeared over, but I had an important question. 'What was the diagnosis?' I asked. The answer was a blow! Our daughter was schizophrenic. We asked whether we should tell our relatives and friends. Should we tell Elizabeth? Should we keep it a secret? 'What kind of life lies ahead for our daughter? Will she be able to go back to school? What about boyfriends and marriage?' we wondered aloud. Most of these questions were not comprehensively answered. However, we were advised to keep the nature of the illness to ourselves. Elizabeth was not to be informed about the diagnosis yet. At my insistence, she would become an outpatient at the same hospital and visit her psychiatrist for a brief interview whenever she needed a new prescription. If there was a chance of repeated illness, I certainly wanted a psychiatrist to be seeing her. And so, virtually uninformed and totally mystified, we brought Elizabeth home to live with us and to a job at a sheltered workshop.

To our surprise we found Elizabeth much easier to live with than she had ever been before. Like an obedient child, compliant and dependent, she carried out all orders, took her medication regularly, and was conscientious about her duties at the workshop. We looked after her, not expecting her to contribute much to the work around the house.

But living with Elizabeth was like living with a robot, and we became increasingly concerned. We looked for an explanation of her condition and blamed both the shock therapy and the medication. Perhaps if the medication was reduced she would be less sluggish, less childlike, we thought. We were, however, in a dilemma since we did not want the drugs decreased at the risk of her illness returning.

Our younger daughter begged us to make an appointment with the psychiatrist. We agreed with her that we should find out the long-term implications of her sister's behavior. We had important questions: Could the medication be reduced? Was there an alternative to the sheltered workshop? Was there a group home that she might eventually move into?

Unfortunately the meeting between Elizabeth's doctor and my husband turned out to be a great disappointment. Elizabeth was on a mere maintenance dose that could not be reduced further and it was best for her to continue at the workshop and to live with us, he advised. The implication was that the situation was not likely to improve ever, and for the first time we felt a growing despair about the future.

However, two or three things happened about this same time that brought dramatic changes to Elizabeth's life.

First, our younger daughter Pamela and her little girl came to live with us, filling our house with activity and giving Elizabeth other young people to mix with and some baby-sitting responsibility. Furthermore, Pamela chided us once more about our complacency. She felt Elizabeth needed a more stimulating atmosphere to live in. We were treating her like a retarded person by keeping her too dependent. She sensed that Elizabeth was at a standstill at the workshop. She made arrangements with her father to have Elizabeth work in his office and trained her in the evenings to do jobs that she could easily manage. She urged us to see another psychiatrist to get a second opinion about Elizabeth's potential for a more independent life.

The second significant occurrence was the change of Elizabeth's doctor. The new psychiatrist was an immediate hit and we were delighted when he invited us to have an interview with him to discuss Elizabeth's progress and to ask questions and make suggestions. Two years after Elizabeth's discharge from hospital we went back for a meeting with him and a psychiatric nurse. It was a marvelous encounter with warm, concerned, and understanding professionals. We were immensely excited and optimistic!

That momentous meeting generated a number of changes in our lives, which in turn contributed to a marked improvement in Elizabeth's behavior. Among other things, Elizabeth enrolled in a special clinic, and my husband and I joined a relatives' group. I must emphasize how beneficial both these connections have been and continue to be for all of us.

Gradually there was a tremendous change in Elizabeth. She began to walk down the street faster, she became more interested in her personal appearance, she began to help around the house, and she went out more. It was as though she were coming back to life.

Last summer she took a trip to Venezuela to visit a former high-school friend and her husband. We were worried about the trip and the change in eating and sleeping patterns, but we had to let her go! She had planned the trip and saved the money for it totally on her own. She had an exciting time and arrived home in great shape.

This last year has brought further change. Less compliant, more self-assured, she is ready to challenge us and to argue and stand up for her rights. Just recently a friend of ours, who had not seen Elizabeth for a year, remarked on the unbelievable change. She commented on her composure, her liveliness, and her contribution to the conversation.

The spectacular change in our daughter was not the result of medication change. Undoubtedly it was tied in with good professional help and a more stimulating atmosphere at work and home.

However, after five years, there still remains the challenge of trying to help Elizabeth become much more independent. She cannot really do that while she works for her father and lives with us. She is now beginning to ask about other jobs and about the necessary training for them. We are exploring the possibilities of a group home. With the support of the clinic and the relatives' group, we think these goals can be accomplished. We are optimistic about Elizabeth's future.

ELEVEN

A father's account

My daughter called from Ottawa, Ontario, one day to say, 'Please send money.' She had gone on a two-day trip and taken $200.00. We couldn't see that she would need more. 'It's very important,' she said, 'a very important person is interested in me.' This sounded odd but, at first, believable. That was the main problem when she first started getting sick: we didn't know if it was make-believe, if she was teasing us, if she was angry at us, or if she was just confused. We quickly realized that it was no fun for her. Her so-called adventures with movie stars and Hollywood producers and politicians and royalty were not making her happy and left her upset all the time. Was she under too much stress at school? we wondered. Was I as a parent responsible for this upset in my child and, if so, in what way? How could I help her face up to reality and accept responsibility for her increasingly inappropriate behavior? Not knowing what to do, we tried to write it off as a passing phase, something she would outgrow, and we did nothing.

As reasoning with her became more and more impossible, it all became too much to cope with – for her and for me, too. Finally, at the end of our patience, we had to turn to professionals for help, but it took us *five years* to realize she had an illness!

Then we were told she had to go to a hospital. This was incredibly upsetting to us, but we had no choice. Her behavior was impossible to control by then. She had dropped out of school, wouldn't look for work, stayed in bed all day, went out at night, and came back with these extraordinary stories. When she was in hospital there was an initial sense of relief that she might now get the help she needed. Then came the shock: we were told that the diagnosis was schizophrenia. They tried to explain what that meant, but it's not an easy thing for a parent to grasp. The main treatment recommended seemed to be drug therapy and we were against that somehow. We didn't know much about schizophrenia then.

I think we weren't alone in having unrealistic expectations about what psychiatry could do and how our child should be treated. I think professionals don't spend nearly enough time explaining, reassuring, and supporting parents. Much of what we learned came by guesswork.

Education of parents and family members about schizophrenia is crucial. Meeting other relatives in a similar position as ourselves is also needed. We found we had to go after assistance, keeping our ears tuned to all sources. Nobody thought to refer us for this kind of help.

Our daughter's problems are not gone. But we are much better informed and know better how to cope with situations as they arise. When she says Prince Charles is courting her, we know it isn't an attention-getting device or a piece of silliness or a maneuver to get more money from us or a deliberate ploy to drive us crazy. That's what we used to think. We realize now that that is how her mind works. When she's feeling down she will try anything to get her spirits up, I think. Now when she says Prince Charles is interested in her, we don't quarrel with her. We don't avoid her either, as we had started to do when we thought she was crazy. We tell her we're interested in her and we make little attempts to make her feel better about herself. It seems to work.

TWELVE

I am a schizophrenic

My name is Sandra. I was diagnosed as a schizophrenic 11 years ago, at the age of 25. Until then I had danced professionally in various nightclubs and, at one point, taught ballet.

In the course of my illness, I went from being a dancer pursued by millionaires and movie stars, to a divorcee working part-time selling two-dollar earrings, and then on to welfare, before I was able to start picking myself up again.

I am now, thanks to treatment and support, a psychiatric nurse, helping people diagnosed as I am, and many others as well. I graduated from nursing three years ago, standing first in my class, with an overall average of 86 percent.

You will notice the title I have given this chapter is "I *am* a schizophrenic" and not I *was* a schizophrenic. Like an alcoholic who has to stand up at a meeting of Alcoholics Anonymous and admit, "I *am* an alcoholic," so I have come to regard schizophrenia as something that is always with me, although not always in a troublesome way.

I would like to take this opportunity to discuss the feelings one experiences in coming to terms with schizophrenia, and show how psychiatry has helped me, in the hope that many will realize that they are not alone, and that when you're 'down' the only way is 'up'!

Understanding schizophrenia

It is not easy to understand an illness like schizophrenia that brings you to a psychiatric facility for help. We are quite prepared to accept the fact we may have a sore arm or aching leg, but how does one accept the fact one has a 'sore' head? For the older set, there was a movie *Snake Pit*, which portrayed Olivia de Havilland locked up, with the key thrown away. Or for the younger set, *One Flew over the Cuckoo's Nest* brought a new sort of fear – lobotomies and shock treatments.

The illness makes us enter a new world, with the possibility of our clothes being taken away from us, or the door being locked for a time to detain us. In most cases we do not realize that it is for our own protection.

We are faced with fears. 'I'm scared for I've never experienced anything like this.'

Some of us feel relieved. 'Home was such hell; this place is like heaven; it's no hassle.'

There are feelings about prior hospitalizations such as 'I feel like a failure when I have to come here. To enter the hospital every few years is something I can't cope with. When I come back, I know I haven't made it.' Or thoughts like, 'I spent six months on a violent ward. I remember another patient slugging me. It was scary, and I thought this place might be the same way.'

All these thoughts are a hindrance to understanding our illness.

Then there is medication. How does one accept the necessity of having to take medication for a long time, especially when it can make you feel unable to think, or shaky and nervous, or like pacing up and down endlessly.

And to add insult to injury, we are told 'You are schizophrenic.' How does one accept this when one has seen the movie *Three Faces of Eve?* I don't know about Joanne Woodward, but I have always had only one personality, although when I was first told that I was a schizophrenic, you can bet your life I spent a lot of idle time trying to find my other personalities.

Yes, we all have fears, some real and some imaginary, and they take time to disappear.

And what about the stigma of being in a psychiatric facility? 'Are my friends going to find out?' 'Is my boss going to find out?' 'If I tell anybody where I was, they might think I'm crazy.'

This brings on another fear: 'I must be "crazy," or why would I be here?'

So how does one understand? Well, by talking about how we feel and by asking questions, reading about the illness, and sharing experiences.

Because of the fears, it took me a long time to understand my illness. I never read, thought no one could possibly understand how I felt, especially the nurses and doctors, for they have never been through this. But through reassurance, comfort, and talking, I realized that there are a lot of people who do understand. Even though maybe they haven't been through the actual illness, they have all been through some traumatic experiences.

Accepting the illness

During my ninth hospitalization (this by itself should tell you how long it took me to accept my illness), I remember writing a poem about the ward I was on. I was very proud of myself as it was put on the bulletin board for everyone to read. I do not remember the poem anymore; however, one line really sticks out in my memory: 'I'm not crazy – they are,' referring to my friends around me. How I denied the fact that I needed help!

Denial is perhaps the worst phase of this illness to go through, and the most costly in time. My average length of stay in hospital was from six to eight weeks, and I was hospitalized nine times. I thus wasted a year and a half of my life denying the fact that I was schizophrenic. How did I do it? – by going off medication as soon as I felt well. How I hated that medication! Every time I took it it was a constant reminder that something was wrong with me, and I hated to think that something was wrong with me.

Every time I was hospitalized, I was told the same thing: 'If you'd stay on the medication, and see your therapist, you probably wouldn't have to be in hospital.' But how I hated to take that medication!

I started to ponder this on my last admission. 'The medication must work. It gets me well enough to get out of here.' 'Do I want to keep on being hospitalized the rest of my life?' 'Maybe I should stay on the medication; I'm not sick, however, it must do something.'

During my last stay in hospital, I was made to confront my denial. I came to accept the fact, through much psychotherapy, that I was schizophrenic, and during my last week in hospital, I was one of three people chosen to talk to over 200 medical students. I remember getting up on that stage and the doctor who was conducting the seminar asking 'Sandra, what is your problem?' I promptly answered, 'I am schizophrenic.' It didn't hurt. In fact I was proud, as I had come to terms with my illness. Five years later – nursing school, a nursing career – it still doesn't hurt.

Friends and relatives

It has been my experience that friends and relatives come in four varieties:

The indifferent ones (or the 'duty' ones)
These are the ones who come to bring you cigarettes when you're in hospital, ask you how you feel, and go on to discuss their own problems. (They do the same when you're not in hospital.)

This hurts. If anyone needs comfort and reassurance, it's us. We're going through hell, you know. Try to understand what's happening to us. We feel weak, vulnerable, and very mixed up. Don't think just because we're safe in the hospital, it's over – it's not. We have to wrestle with every feeling, thought, and emotion we are feeling; and it's not easy.

The overprotective ones

These are the ones who see us as 'invalids.' We can't do anything anymore. We should just stay home, rest, and be babied. Quit school, give up our jobs, et cetera. *Don't*, please don't do this. Accept the fact we're a little helpless now but not hopeless.

I remember speaking to a group of schizophrenics who were meeting with their parents. One of the parents was fearful about taking his daughter on a six-week trip to Europe. 'It would be too much of a strain.' I was furious! Don't make us feel any worse! Encourage activities we were once doing. If you don't accept us, who will?

The fearful type

'Well, he's crazy now, better stay away from him.' This hurts. How do you expect us to get well if you won't accept we are ill and can get better with help? It makes *us* deny we are ill even more, and it's very lonely, being 'alone.'

The honest type

They are at first as bewildered as the other types but they are obviously trying to learn about the illness, both from us and from others. They are constantly looking for answers to problems and questions, both on their own as well as with us.

Hospitalization (the team)

I remember one of my most frustrating concerns as a patient: 'How can I expect to get well when I never see the doctor?' As with every other patient, my doctor knew everything, no one else did, and he, and he alone, could help. I never understood the importance of psychologists, social workers, occupational therapists, or nurses. I only wanted to see my doctor, and could never understand why he wasn't at my beck and call.

Now that I am a nurse, I would like to introduce you to 'The

Team,' with the doctor as head of the team. Why a team? The doctor has many patients and he cannot spend all his time with you. So all the members of his team act as mini-doctors by listening to you, helping you grasp your problems, and guiding you towards a solution to your problems. As team members we all write notes or inform the doctor in person of how you are doing, and he makes the decisions as a result of the team's effort to help you. So do not feel you are being ignored. Many are working for you. And many are much more approachable and understanding and helpful than the doctor.

Boring the therapist

As a patient and as a nurse, I have come to realize there is no such thing in psychiatry as boring the therapist. Everything one says helps the therapist understand what the patient is all about. And by helping him realize what we are all about, he can in turn help *us* realize what it is that bothers us about ourselves. Take my own case for example.

I see my psychiatrist on the average every two weeks or once a month. In examining what I am 'all about,' it became clear that many of my symptoms crop up when I am rejected by members of the opposite sex. My doctor and I now spend our therapy sessions mainly discussing the men I know and how I react to them. I used to feel I was wasting her time talking about things that I thought would be better discussed with a girlfriend, but I have realized that this is part of the treatment that keeps me well.

It is very important to take responsibility for raising problems and for working at one's difficulties. Being honest and direct with therapists helps a great deal.

Expecting the world to look after you

As I explained earlier, I went from being a dancer pursued by millionaires and movie stars to a divorcee selling two-dollar earrings, and then to being on welfare. Part of the reason for my difficulties was that I felt sorry for myself. 'Why am I sick? Why am I always in hospital? Why aren't my friends in hospital? Why aren't my family?' Expecting the world to look after you is again a form of DENIAL. It is denying the fact that we feel alone, helpless and hopeless, that we need help, that we're sick and many other things.

Don't let this happen to you. TALK ABOUT how you feel. DON'T REMAIN ALONE. Join activities, see your doctor or therapist, tell them how you feel. Again, don't feel nobody understands. It is natural to feel sorry for yourself at one point, but don't stay 'down.' Being 'down' is degrading financially, physically, and emotionally. Feeling helpless makes one feel hopeless; having hope brings help. The medical profession will always offer help even if friends and relatives don't, so accept it.

Don't give up!

I recall how I was starting to give up. Looking back now I can genuinely say that it was my own fault. I NEVER UNDERSTOOD the fact that help was there. I kept thwarting it by not accepting that the medical profession knew more than I. 'No one could possibly know or understand what I was going through.' I never understood that I was denying the illness that for several years brought me so much misery; I never understood that I was not capable of coping with many problems on my own. I never appreciated that many of my hospitalizations were my own fault. In other words, I never understood MYSELF, and half the battle in getting well is getting to know yourself.

So, get to know yourself! Get to know that most of the emotions we feel are normal, and that we all have problems and have to learn to talk about them and to understand them, and then to cope with them.

THIRTEEN

A schizophrenic's story

Have you ever woken up realizing that something is seriously wrong, and you don't know if it is physical or mental?

Well this happened to me. I thought that I was going to have a heart attack: the pounding in my chest was ceaseless, my head was spinning. I couldn't think or do anything. All I could do was lie there and suffer. This was the beginning of my breakdown, brought about by several things. A workaholic, worrying all the time, I was slowly losing touch with reality, preferring instead to daydream all the time.

I phoned a psychiatrist whom I had seen a few times the year before. I tried, through screaming and crying, to explain that something had definitely gone wrong with me over the past year. He recommended that I come to the hospital. I agreed, and that became one of several admissions to a psychiatric ward.

Immediately after being admitted, the relief that flowed through my veins slowly relaxed my mind, but I also went back to my fantasy world. I was psychotic, but it was the rest of the world that was at fault. I fooled everyone except myself. On discharge I took a vacation in California. The whole time I was away I couldn't face the reality of having been psychotic. More and more I would retreat to the living hell in my mind. I was feeling terribly guilty about everything I had thought and done for 20 years. I was talking to myself and crying and laughing all at the same time. I was thinking that the only way out of this hell was to be violent, not only to myself but to those around me too. I hated myself and my loved ones, but most of all I hated the world. I became increasingly listless and withdrawn, locking myself in my room for days at a time. I had to make a decision: either kill myself or hurt someone or get help. I decided to get help.

I went on day care this time. I was taking Valium and Stelazine just to be able to get up in the morning, but when my psychiatrist took me off Valium I went through hell for two weeks: convulsions, vomiting, diarrhea, and no appetite at all. Other tranquilizers and antidepressants did not help. The doctor couldn't figure out what was wrong. He guessed that I might have a form of schizophrenia but he didn't tell me. Instead he transferred me to a psychiatric hospital for the more intensive care I needed. My new doctor told me that he was not yet sure of the diagnosis, but that I was very sick. When he stopped all medication, I felt angry. I wasn't sleeping, and I was hallucinating. While lying on one bed I could actually *see* myself getting up out of another bed. I was hearing strange people whispering words into my ears. My doctor then told me that I had a form of schizophrenia. He put me on increasing doses of chlorpromazine. It slowed my thinking down and had a calming effect but it didn't take away my violent thoughts. I realized that it was time for me to face the reality of my situation and start to deal with it. I couldn't just sit there with my thoughts and expect the staff and drugs to cure me. That is only 10 percent of it. What people with mental illness must first realize is that most of the cure or control of mental illness is up to the patient. If you want to get better badly enough, you will. The longer you sit and do nothing, the longer it will take to get better. In fact, you may get worse. At first I didn't believe it, but deep down inside, I had the desire and motivation to better myself. What I needed was a spark to get going. In my case they used reverse psychology, which caused me to rely less and less upon feeling sorry for myself and more and more on both co-operating (not conforming) with the staff and listening to how other patients felt and talked. Soon I realized that I wasn't as badly off as I had thought. There were other patients who didn't have a friend or family to speak to. I found myself wanting to talk to them more and more. This was a new beginning for me. I was finally listening to what someone else had to say. I had not cried for a whole year until then. I was still having problems with not being able to think straight.

A change of medication did not help me to straighten it out. This is when I began electroconvulsive therapy (ECT). The first treatment, of a total of 18, gave me a headache. I received these treatments Monday, Wednesday, and Friday mornings over a period of six weeks. Although I had thought of it as a rather grisly form of treatment, it actually worked on me. It slowed down my thinking to normal speed and, together with a drug called pericyazine (Neuleptil), actually helped me to reorganize my unsorted mind.

The next step was psychotherapy. This was a heated and mind-blowing experience. My doctor was basically trying to help me help myself, but I continued to have violent thoughts to the point of being afraid to light a cigarette for fear of setting the ward on fire. Despite those periods of irrationality I was slowly regaining stability and strength. One day my defensive wall finally came down. I was so angry and upset I wanted to both hit my doctor and break down and cry. I did the latter: it was my first relief in more than a year. Rather than accepting my anger early on, I used to deny to the end that I was angry at anyone.

The next week my doctor informed me that I would be discharged in three weeks. With no place to live and no future to speak of, I felt I had to do something to enable me to stay on in hospital. The old anxiety returned, my head was aching, and the violent thoughts became stronger and I started to withdraw again. I pleaded that I was still crazy and a danger to myself.

My social worker, whom I still love as I love my family, gave me a tremendous amount of support. She explained to me about life in a group home, which is a home where people who have had emotional and mental problems live together and share day-to-day problems. There are also problems that arise as the result of living with 10 other people under the same roof. The fact that some may still be slightly ill can be depressing to someone who is trying to climb the ladder of accomplishment again. It is a reminder of one's immediate past. The good thing about it is that it pushes you to try harder to help yourself.

My social worker helped me find a group home two weeks before discharge. We went there during the evening and were welcomed very warmly. I thought to myself that maybe this is the place to make another start in life.

In the hospital I had just completed the program in rehabilitation testing. The tests showed that I was intelligent and could be whatever I wanted to be. They asked me if I would like to take a college course in job-readiness training. I was terrified at first. I would fail and become a lost cause. But I am a fighter and accepted the offer.

I was discharged on a Saturday to the group home and couldn't sleep. I was too excited by this adventure. On Sunday I joined everyone in the dining room for dinner, fearful that I would end up as a welfare bum like many others, having $12 a month spending money, the rest going towards room and board. Right there I decided I would give life a good shot.

Monday morning I returned to the hospital as a day-care patient from 9 am to 4 pm. I was seeing my doctor on a regular basis and was revealing things that had lived within me for years. Whatever I did, one priority had to be dealing with reality, life, death, success, failure. These things I had never experienced. I had merely 'survived.' I was experiencing emotions like never before. They were bad and good feelings, feelings of hate, love, compassion, needing to be with people, and a general desire to live!

The first problem in therapy is trust in your doctor. People are afraid to reveal intimate secrets to people they don't know, preferring instead to feel ashamed or guilty, afraid that if they confide in him he will not like them and maybe even reject them.

A week after discharge I started the school course. My closest friends from the group home also started on that day. It helped reduce the feeling of insecurity and helped to create a common bond.

It was during this time that I felt a need to really express myself. I thought that maybe if I'd write down my feelings on paper I wouldn't feel so depressed. I wrote my first poem called 'Problems.' It was to be my way of coping with reality. I know this sounds strange, but I felt inspired to write it. Even today I look at it from time to time to remind myself that there is hope not only for myself but for everyone else.

School was really having an effect on my life. Just getting up early every morning was a pleasure instead of a job. I was receiving a Manpower allowance to support myself, and things appeared to be going quite well. But I had a problem with drinking. Let's face it: I was once again avoiding reality. I felt under pressure and this was my way of easing it. Not only did I know that I was jeopardizing my future, but I couldn't afford it. My girlfriend was lending me money so I could drink. (Two years later I just said to myself that this had to stop, so I stopped it.)

On finishing the course my closest friend and I enrolled in another course designed to give us a career. It was called industrial production orientation and was a real drag.

It was coming into summer when we graduated, so we both enrolled in a trade course called appliance servicing. This was a one-year trade course. I was afraid I wouldn't last through the year. I gave it a good shot though and, yes, I graduated. My friend today repairs microwave ovens and is a master at it! I never did find a job in my trade.

Living in the group home was getting a little tough to deal with because as I was getting better the other people in the home seemed to be getting worse. I found this hard to deal with. I decided to stay there until my education was completed.

My doctor and I would sit down for one hour a week discussing and trying to solve my problems. It took one and a half years to control my violent thoughts, yet I would deny that I was angry with anyone. Actually I was very angry at the world for what I felt was a bad deal I got in life. The violent thoughts were my way of dealing with that feeling. Actually when I faced the truth it really hurt. I wasn't really given such a bad deal in life. Life has its ups and its downs. One must learn how to deal with it. I shed a lot of tears while going through this pain. My doctor would not feed into my feeling sorry for myself. It's okay to feel sorry for yourself, but don't prolong it. You've got to go on living your life, and feeling sorry for yourself for a long period could prevent you from doing anything about your life. He was really tough on me. He would not let me get away with denying anything. Honesty with a doctor is the best policy. I found that out.

I wish I could write that I have been successful, but I can't. My thoughts are better and I feel better, but I am poor, haven't got a job yet, and will be going to school again. But I haven't given up!

FOURTEEN

A mother's point of view

The beginning: not understanding

As a parent of a child developing symptoms of schizophrenia, you cannot understand what is happening. For a long time we thought our son's strange behavior was due to street drugs, so we tried to handle it with discipline. We feel now that he was sick long before the drugs. What we realize now is that the marijuana temporarily made him feel better: that's why he used it.

The main question in our minds now is how come we had so little knowledge? As a mother, I did not need a doctor to tell me my children had measles or any other fairly common illness. I had taken first aid courses. I had read about health care. Why did I never come across articles on schizophrenia or other mental illnesses that affect young people? With something that is so serious and touches so many people, why the secret? I will never understand why mental illnesses are not as widely publicized as any other illnesses.

The acute attack: not knowing what to do

Our son had taken a small amount of LSD and was acting what we thought was very scared. We called our family doctor, who sug-

gested calling a psychiatric hospital. When they heard about the
LSD, the hospital told us to go to the addiction center. We did and
followed instructions: 24 hours a day of supervised home care, no
street drugs, and twice-weekly visits to the doctor. After six weeks
of this, our son was getting worse instead of better. The doctor then
arranged for his entry into the psychiatric hospital.

Finding the right doctor

Finding a good doctor in any field is very difficult. With so many
of the doctors treating mental disorders having so many different
views about everything, a good psychiatrist is hard to find. Nothing
is worse than talking to someone who avoids your questions. Then
you always imagine the worst. It was a relief finally to have a
doctor who sat down with us and was honest about my son's
condition. He answered all our questions and yet left us with lots of
hope.

The family's reaction

When a member of the family becomes disturbed like this, a sort of
shock sets in at first. You withdraw from friends, not from shame
but from a hurt so deep you cannot talk about it. You cannot
understand, so how can you hope to have others understand? You
don't want to talk about it but you can think of nothing else. Tears
run down the face of a husband who never cries, and a wife who
cries for any small reason cannot, now when it might help. At this
early stage there is no humor in the world.

When he was hospitalized, it was a very sad time, but at least
now we felt he was getting the help he needed so badly. Our own
lives were finally able to start again.

How we deal with things in the family now

I try to encourage our son on the good days to get the most out of them. We talk about his day and all the good things he can do and enjoy. On the bad days (we expect there will be many) we want him to understand that they are not a major setback but only a period that will pass. He must get to understand the illness well enough to ignore the bad days and to carry on.

We never lie to our son because we want him to trust us. Our son is not treated as if he were ill. He is an important member of the family with equal rights. We expect him to be well-groomed, respectful, cheerful if possible, and to try to improve. We expect him to let us know when something is wrong and to tell us how he is feeling. We have many days when we enjoy his company very much.

You can't tell someone with schizophrenia what to do: you can only encourage. We make no big deal about medicine. If I am not too demanding or too critical, he is usually easy to get along with.

How a relative's group has helped

I have developed a good understanding of the problems of medication and lack of motivation of the average schizophrenic person. I understand some of the problems of group homes, boarding homes, and the difficult family situations of some patients and families. I know something about services available in the community. I think I have a basic knowledge of some of the symptoms of the illness which are fairly normal and when we should seek help. I realize you cannot push a schizophrenic. You take each day at a time and you enjoy the good things. You encourage and praise and gently ease things until they are better. The illness seems to go up and down. As parents, we should stay cool and try to keep our family life as normal as possible. You must not allow yourself to become discouraged. I feel families with similar problems can help each other. I would like to help other families as confused as we were to understand how to live a life as normal as possible in spite of the problems of schizophrenia.

Eleven points to remember

1 Never give up; things always improve.
2 Guilt complexes (trying to figure out what you did wrong) are a waste of time. It happened; get on with where you go from here.
3 Do things that make *you* happy.
4 Remember your child is *ill*. He can't help his illness any more than he could if he were paralyzed. Try to keep this in mind. Be patient.
5 Grooming can be a problem, but try to be positive. Tell him how handsome he is when well-groomed. Leave good clothes handy; hide the old scruffy things he may insist on wearing. Leave shampoo handy and be sure to comment on his clean hair.
6 Encourage his friends to phone or drop in.
7 Never put your son down. He has heard enough of that. Never try to hide him from friends or relatives.
8 Hold on to your religious beliefs; you really need them. (I think this point should be near the top of the list.)
9 Read and seek out all the information you can on your child's illness. Go to mental health lectures put on by mental health associations. Attend lectures at your hospital. Don't hesitate to ask your child's doctor any questions, no matter how ridiculous you think they may sound.
10 Above all, love your child when he is at his worst. Don't wait for him to fulfill your expectations.
11 Take one day at a time. Don't try to solve problems a year or 10 years from now.

FIFTEEN

The doctor's dilemma

Schizophrenia is a serious illness and involves a long, hard struggle for the patient and those around him. The doctor to whom the care of a patient is assigned has to deal with situations that can at times be very difficult. The real task is to maintain realistic hopefulness in the face of frustrating setbacks and never to 'give up' on a patient. I know that many of my actions are perceived as unwelcome or unpleasant, even though they are intended to help.

My view of schizophrenia obviously determines how I approach care and treatment. I consider schizophrenia a severe disturbance of the brain chemistry, producing very unusual and sometimes frightening experiences. This is the physical, biological basis of the illness. The way one reacts to the psychotic experience is the psychological component. Most people react with fright and mystification at the strangeness of it and at the implication that this is 'crazy.' They are also influenced by the reactions of family, friends, and colleagues.

In my training period I was taught that to be a good psychiatrist one had to be able to understand how the patient felt, for this was the basis of 'therapy'; I was told, however, that it was difficult to relate to schizophrenia patients because they have problems in developing relationships. The implication was: 'Don't bother trying.' I see things differently now. I perceive that the patient has suffered a terrible trauma: the loss of sanity, which we all take so much for granted. No wonder schizophrenics feel sad and hopeless and lose their zest for life; no wonder they become afraid to face others, afraid that somehow their madness, their 'difference,' will be seen by others! What a blow to their self-esteem and their self-confidence, particularly so when the illness strikes just as people are making plans for the future, for jobs, and for social and sexual relationships. I can understand that patients will be afraid of me, afraid of being treated primarily as 'mad,' their personhood, their humanity, a distant second. They have every good reason to meet me cautiously.

And what of me? How on earth can I really understand what it is like to be 'mad,' 'crazy,' psychotic? I became aware of my own fear of madness and how it inclined me to keep my distance. This realization has influenced all my subsequent work. There was a subtle change in my thinking from considering my patients as 'schizophrenics' to realizing that they were people, just like me, but afflicted with the illness schizophrenia. I relate to all the people I meet who have schizophrenia as individuals. I want a personal relationship with them, and I want them to have a personal relationship with me. Then, together, we can get down to the business of treating their illness.

As a psychiatrist, I know that the best way of dealing with the biological basis of schizophrenia is by the well-adjusted intake of medication (neuroleptics). I also know that the medication I prescribe has its side-effects, at times quite troublesome, and I have to be sensitive to the patient's reports of such side-effects. I know that few people relish the idea of having to carry on with treatment procedures ad infinitum. Whether one thinks of schizophrenia, or arthritis, or allergies, or dialysis for kidney failure, the obligation to carry on with a treatment day after day for weeks and months and years is often seen as demoralizing, especially by young people. Not surprisingly there is a tendency to rebel from time to time against such an indefinite treatment regime. I have to admit that I sympathize with the motives for stopping treatment. At the same time I owe it to my patients to urge them to continue with long-term treatment.

This creates conflict between my patients and me. I would like to illustrate the dilemma and its resolution by talking about some patients, the first in some detail.

My first contact with Grace dates back seven years; at that time she already had had eight years of intense, severe psychosis, starting at the age of 22. I reviewed her chart and noted that she had spent 38 of the previous 94 months as an inpatient. She had had 12 admissions, some as brief as three days, others as long as 12 months. She had had her longest stay out of hospital (a period of 18 months) while being treated with a long-acting injectable antipsychotic medication. She was difficult to treat. A pattern developed wherein she would respond very slowly to medication, would get well after a long struggle, have a period of remission, stop her medication, and soon become ill again. Even when taking medication, she was susceptible to depressive episodes.

By the time I started to work with her, she was 29 years old. Her father had died when she was 18, and her mother, who had deserted the family when Grace was only 9, was at that time chronically ill and hospitalized because of multiple sclerosis. Grace was seen by many of the hospital staff as permanently impaired at the time she was referred to me for treatment. She had been told by other doctors to avoid all stress because it might lead to a breakdown. Above all, she had been told not to develop any close relationships with the opposite sex because these were sure to produce a breakdown. It had also been suggested that work was likely to be too much of a stress. For a number of years she had been treated by a psychiatrist who showed a great deal of warmth and interest, but she had developed a childlike, dependent attitude towards him. It became clear to her early on that she was not going to have the same type of relationship with me. Although I had genuine interest and concern for her, I also wanted her to be as independent as possible. Perhaps I risk being disappointed when I set expectations of independence, but I feel it is better to err on the side of too high rather than too low a standard. With Grace I was agreeably surprised because it soon appeared that she was capable of taking on a good deal of responsibility for herself and becoming fairly self-sufficient. She soon learned a great deal about her illness.

After two years we got into a series of disagreements. Grace kept requesting reductions in her medication. Since she did not have any side-effects, I tended to resist her requests, but from time to time I found myself going along with her wishes saying, 'Well, we'll take a chance. We'll just have to wait and see how it turns out.' Then I realized that whenever she made these requests she was refusing to accept the reality of her illness. She was hoping that somehow it would just go away and that she would not need the medication. It seemed impossible to convince her, though I continued to try. Another considerable source of worry for me was that at times she thought longingly of being psychotic again. Certain components of a psychosis can appear attractive: the freedom to do the bizarre and the seeming freedom from responsibility. Eventually it came to a confrontation between Grace and me. She wanted me to take her off medication, and I said that I could not do this and still fulfill my responsibility as her doctor.

I had moments of self-doubt; perhaps she was right about the medication and about my being too conservative and my anticipating the return of her psychosis where none actually threatened; perhaps, too, it was cruel of me to continue to urge her towards 'health' when madness might be less of a struggle.

In fact she stopped her medication on her own and became psychotic a few months later, a pattern that has recurred since. Is insanity a 'reasonable' option that people should be free to choose?

Harry is a 35-five-year-old man whose schizophrenia had been diagnosed late because his personality difficulties and drug abuse clouded the picture. With him, every drug I prescribed he reported as causing serious side-effects without much objective evidence. Clearly he did not like taking any of the neuroleptic drugs. On one occasion he insisted upon hospitalization, threatening serious harm to himself and others if I refused to admit him to the ward. It was clear that there was some conflict in his life that he was trying to resolve in this manner, but strenuous attempts on my part to clarify these issues with him were unsuccessful. I was afraid that he would act on his threats if I did not accede to his request for hospitalization.

He was discharged after only one week, but I worried about the future with this man who does not accept medication but who has proved he can 'blackmail' me into hospitalizing him. On other occasions Harry has attempted to deal with the conflict between us by asking for a referral to another doctor. He makes initial contact with other physicians, but invariably returns to see me. I often feel that I am fighting a losing battle. To help him remain well, I need to prescribe medication that he is not willing to take. He thus remains unwell, in my care but not under my treatment.

What is the doctor to do under these circumstances? I am never sure how tough to be. One young man, Jim, did poorly during a prolonged hospitalization. We discovered this was because he was smoking marijuana both off and on the ward. Restricting him to the ward and monitoring his visitors led to a marked recovery though it gave the staff the nasty responsibility of being 'jailers.' When he improved, we discussed the dangers of marijuana and he was again allowed off the ward only to return speedily to marijuana use and a flare-up of his schizophrenia. Frustrated, we decided to restrict him again, but this time he would not accept the restrictions and left the hospital and the city. Naturally his illness flared within a few days and he was returned to us, still unwilling to give up his marijuana use.

The marijuana abuse presents a threat to other patients who may be given it by Jim; it also makes the staff feel powerless, and when they feel powerless they get angry at me. Should I discharge the patient and face the wrath of the family, or keep him longer, trying to treat him with the aid of an unsympathetic staff? This is one of those tricky situations where I can please the patient by ordering his discharge while angering his family.

Some conflicts turn out well. A patient with whom I had had a warm, collaborative relationship became acutely ill. The family was unable to cope; the patient did not see himself as ill but actually presented a considerable risk to his own safety. I decided to commit the patient to the hospital. He insisted that he would never trust me again. Should 1 go ahead and risk losing the relationship? Or should I go along with the patient and risk a worsening of the illness and possible harm to the patient or to others? I almost felt like a traitor but I did admit the patient involuntarily. He didn't speak to me at first but, as he improved, he realized what had happened and understood his illness better than before. My action actually cemented our relationship.

Sometimes my own staff may disagree with me about treatment. For example, some of the staff are reluctant to make use of ECT, which I believe to be an effective and humane treatment for certain conditions. It is difficult to proceed with any treatment plan or therapy without staff cohesiveness, so that much time needs to be spent in team conferences and discussions. Patients are quick to sense staff disagreements, and it is often under these circumstances that they refuse treatment.

Patients and their families sometimes seem to get the impression that we doctors have a set treatment approach from which we do not deviate, and that we are not sensitive to their concerns and suggestions. Clearly for a doctor to behave like that is poor medicine. We cannot always act exactly in accordance with the demands of the patient or family, but we must always be open to their suggestions and willing to incorporate them whenever possible. The central conflict remains: unlike most other illnesses, schizophrenia may affect a person in such a way that he genuinely does not feel in need of treatment.

Schizophrenia presents the physician with many complex problems. It is an area in which relatively few psychiatrists specialize,
partly because of these recurrent dilemmas. I have often pondered
what makes it worthwhile. I can't be really sure but I think for me
it is a deep concern for those affected by this illness. The illness,
schizophrenia, is a common enemy to be conquered. Often it is
unconquerable. Frequently it can only be held at bay, with ultimate
victory, it is to be hoped, somewhere in the future. The psychiatrist
cannot fight it alone. I have come to realize that I need the help of
colleagues skilled in specialized areas, of the individual patients,
and of their families. And victory comes closer when I can convey
to my patient that the struggle is worth it.

Agencies and services

This is an *alphabetical* listing of agencies and services that may prove useful at different stages of the management of schizophrenia. For families moving to new communities, telephone listings for these services may be obtained in telephone directories. Once you have entered into the network of helpful services, you are more likely to be informed when something new and better becomes available.

Academy of Medicine (might be listed under 'M' for medical society or 'P' for physicians and surgeons): The academy of medicine will suggest the names of physicians and psychiatric specialists in your neighborhood. Many psychiatrists subspecialize; for example, they take particular interest in adolescent psychiatry, in family, group, or marital therapy, or in schizophrenia. The academy of medicine may be able to provide information about subspecialization.

Ambulances: Ambulances for transporting ill individuals to hospital are emergency services and are usually listed on the first or second page of the telephone directory.

Associations: Local chapters of medical, psychological, social work, psychiatric, and self-help associations will be listed under 'Associations.'

Consulates: For travelers abroad, your local consulate will inform you of local facilities.

Crisis or distress centers: These are telephone advice services for crisis situations and are usually listed at the front of telephone books.

Drug addiction information and treatment centers: These services are sometimes needed because drug abuse, like alcohol abuse, may become a secondary problem for some people with schizophrenia.

Drug crisis centers: These are detoxification centers for drug and alcohol problems and may be listed under emergency services.

Foundations: These are educational, philanthropic, and research foundations, some of which may be related to work with schizophrenia.

Government services: Everyone should look through the listings under government services for an overview of services provided at the various levels of government. These include income security (family allowances, disability and welfare pensions, unemployment insurance); employment, including handicapped employment; health information and insurance; public health laboratories; mental health centers; psychiatric hospitals; housing; children's services; drug benefits; social services; community centers; legal services (justice of the peace, family law, social work assistance, psychiatric services); coroner's office; police; protection and parole; immigrant reception services; and human rights branches. In the United States the central headquarters for government mental health services is: National Institute of Mental Health, 5600 Fishers Lane, Rockville, Md 20857.

Hospitals: Hospitals may or may not be listed by district. A telephone call to the nearest hospital will provide information about its emergency and psychiatric services. Psychiatric hospitals may be listed separately. A visit to the psychiatric services of different hospitals may help one to decide which setting is most appropriate for a particular person. Health insurance may cover one type of hospital setting and not another. In the United States contact: American Hospital Association, 840 North Lake Shore Drive, Chicago, Ill 60611.

Lawyers and legal services: Lawyers are listed by district. Legal Aid is available in most communities.

Libraries: Municipal, university, and hospital libraries may be a good source of reading material about schizophrenia.

Mental health associations: City, state or provincial, and national mental health associations are active in different communities. In the United States contact: Mental Health Association, National Headquarters, 1800 North Kent Street, Arlington, Va 22209; in Canada: Canadian Mental Health Association, 2160 Yonge Street, Toronto, Ontario M4S 2Z3.

Newspapers: Newspaper articles about new research or new therapeutic programs may direct you to helpful services. Announcements of meetings of local groups, foundations, and associations interested in schizophrenia should be watched for in the local papers. In the United States other publications are available from: Public Inquiries Section, National Clearinghouse for Mental Health Information, National Institute of Mental Health, 5600 Fishers Lane, Rockville, Md 20857.

Nurses: Visiting, public health, and private nurses are available in most communities.

Nursing home placement services: These are available in some communities.

Personal services: Homemaker, maid, babysitting, and companion services are available. These may be required when the family plans a vacation.

Pharmacies: Pharmacists are usually good sources of information about medications and may provide reading material about drugs used in schizophrenia.

Physicians and surgeons: Doctors are listed in telephone directories under this title. There is usually no separate listing for psychiatrists, but the doctor's specialty may be listed after his name. A call to the office will provide information about referral procedure, fees, and the doctor's special interests.

Poison information: In case of overdose, local poison information centers are listed on the first or second page of the telephone directory.

Police: The number for the police is always prominently displayed at the front of the telephone directory.

Radio and television: Science and public service programs are frequently good sources of new information about schizophrenia.

Rehabilitation services: Private services will be listed separately from government-subsidized rehabilitation services.

Religious organizations: Many religious organizations provide hostels, day activity programs, food and clothing supplies to the poor, and counseling services.

Social service organizations: This is an important listing. It includes family and child service agencies, community information services; suicide prevention centers; food, clothing, and shelter for the indigent; housing for special groups, including ex-psychiatric patients; legal services; meals on wheels for shut-ins; translator services for immigrants; self-help groups; and educational services. In the United States write to: The Assembly of National Voluntary Health and Social Welfare Organizations, 345 East 46th Street, New York, NY 10017.

Self-help groups

There are organizations designed especially for ex-psychiatric patients, and some are especially designed for persons with schizophrenia and/or their relatives. The following are some useful addresses, listed alphabetically by country, by state within the United States, and by province within Canada.

Australia

Canberra
Canberra Schizophrenia
  Fellowship, Inc.
Shout Office
Hughes Community Centre
Wisdom St
Hughes 2605
Tel: 062-812-983

New South Wales
Schizophrenia Fellowship of New
  South Wales
C/-8 Dunmore Ave
Carlingford 2118
Tel: 02-882-053

Queensland
Schizophrenia Fellowship of
  Central Queensland
'Leichhardt'
P.O. Box 7, Dysart 4745
Tel: 079-581-252

Schizophrenia Fellowship of
  Northern Queensland
P.O. Box 979
Hermit Park 4812
Tel: 077-752-152

Schizophrenia Fellowship of
  South Queensland
P.O. Box 1567, Brisbane 4001
Queen St
Tel: 07-870-7536-5481
or 07-358-4424

South Australia
Schizophrenia Fellowship of
    South Australia
Mental Health Resource Centre
35 Fullarton Rd
Kent Town 5067
Tel: 08-362-6772

Victoria
Schizophrenia Fellowship of
    Victoria
211 Chapel St, 3rd Floor
Prahran 3181
Tel: 03-521-2433

Schizophrenia Australia
    Foundation
P.O. Box 236
Prahran 3181
Tel: 03-521-2433

Canada

Alberta
Alberta Friends of Schizophrenics
2405–9th Ave S.E., Suite 102
Calgary T2W 1J8
Tel: (404) 262-4554

British Columbia
British Columbia Friends of
    Schizophrenics
2515 Burrard St, Suite 204
Vancouver V6J 3J5
Tel: (604) 734-3613

Manitoba
Manitoba Friends of
    Schizophrenics
4–1000 Notre Dame Ave
Winnipeg R3E 0N3
Tel: (204) 786-1616

Newfoundland
Newfoundland Friends of
    Schizophrenics
Rabbittown Community Centre
28 Graves St
St John's A1B 3C5
Tel: (709) 579-4834

Nova Scotia
Nova Scotia Friends of
    Schizophrenics
P.O. Box 178
Mt Uniacke B0N 1Z0
Tel: (902) 465-2601

Ontario
Canadian Friends of
    Schizophrenics
95 Barber Green Rd, Suite 309
Don Mills M3C 3E9
Tel: (416) 445-8204

Ontario Friends of Schizophrenics
P.O. Box 217, Station 'O'
Toronto M4A 2W3
Tel: (416) 926-1974

Quebec
Quebec Alliance for the
    Mentally Ill Inc.
P.O. Box 145
Station Côte-de-Neiges
Montreal H3S 2S5
Tel: (514) 486-1448

La Fédération québecoise des
   familles et amis du malade
   mental
2270 rue Papineau, bureau 7
Montréal H2K 4J6
Tel: (514) 524-7131

Saskatchewan
Saskatchewan Friends of
   Schizophrenics
Box 305
Regina S4P 3A1
Tel: (306) 584-2620

New Zealand

Schizophrenia Fellowship of
   New Zealand
P.O. Box 593
Christchurch

Republic of Ireland

Schizophrenia Association of
   Ireland
4 Fitzwilliam Pl
Dublin 2
Tel: Dublin 76-1988

United Kingdom

Channel Islands
Jersey Schizophrenia Fellowship
c/o Mrs M. Harrison
Clos du Saie
Rozel, Jersey
Channel Islands
Tel: 0534-51244

England
London Advisory Centre
197 Kings Cross Rd
London WC1X 9BZ
Tel: 01-837-6436

National Schizophrenia
   Fellowship
Midlands Regional Office
9 St Michaels Ct
Victoria St W.
Bromwich B7O 8EZ
Tel: 021-500-5988

Northern Schizophrenia
   Fellowship
38 Collingwood Buildings
Collingwood St
Newcastle-upon-Tyne NE1 1JH
Tel: 091-261-4343

National Schizophrenia
   Fellowship
Southern Regional Office
17 Oxford St
Southampton SO1 1DJ
Tel: 0703-225664

National Schizophrenia
   Fellowship
78 Victoria Rd
Surbiton, Surrey KT6 4NS
Tel: 01-390-3651

Northern Ireland
National Schizophrenia
   Fellowship
47 Rosemary St
Belfast BT1 1QB
Tel: 0232-248006

Scotland
National Schizophrenia
    Fellowship
40 Shandwick Pl
Edinburgh EH2 4RT
Tel: 031-226-2025

Wales
National Schizophrenia
    Fellowship
Pen-y-Fai Hospital
Bridgend, Mid-Glamorgan
CF31 4LN
Tel: 0656-766330

United States

Alaska
Alliance for the Mentally Ill
4050 Lake Otis Pkwy, #103
Anchorage 99508
Tel: (907) 561-3127

Arkansas
Alliance for the Mentally Ill
4313 W. Markham, Rm 233
Little Rock 72201
Tel: (501) 661-1548

California
Alliance for the Mentally Ill
2306 J St, #203
Sacramento 95816
Tel: (916) 443-6417

Colorado
Alliance for the Mentally Ill
1100 Fillmore St
Denver 80206
Tel: (303) 798-1882

Delaware
Alliance for the Mentally Ill
3705 Concord Pike
Wilmington 19803
Tel: (303) 478-3060

District of Columbia
Alliance for the Mentally Ill
422 8th St S.E.
Washington 20003
Tel: (202) 546-0646

Florida
Alliance for the Mentally Ill
400 S. Dixie Hwy, #414
Lake Worth 33460
Tel: (305) 582-1835

Georgia
Alliance for the Mentally Ill
1256 Briarcliffe Rd N.E.
Rm 412–S
Atlanta 30306–2694
Tel: (404) 874-7351

Illinois
Alliance for the Mentally Ill
805 E. Miller St
P.O. Box 4606
Springfield 62708
Tel: (217) 522-1403
or 1-800-346-4572 (in Ill. only)

Indiana
Alliance for the Mentally Ill
Parkview Hospital's South Unit
Lougheed Center
P.O. Box 5624
Ft. Wayne 46895–5624
Tel: (219) 432-4085

Iowa
Alliance for the Mentally Ill
1024 24th St
Box 495
West Des Moines
Tel: (515) 225-8666

Kentucky
Alliance for the Mentally Ill
707 Executive Suite
Louisville 40205
Tel: (502) 896-1877

Louisiana
Alliance for the Mentally Ill
2431 S. Acadian Thruway
Suite 420
Baton Rouge 70808
Tel: (504) 928-6928

Maine
Alliance for the Mentally Ill
2 Union St
Camden 04843
Tel: (207) 236-8047

Maryland
Alliance for the Mentally Ill
2300 N. Charles St
Baltimore 21218
Tel: (301) 235-2511

Massachusetts
Alliance for the Mentally Ill
164 Canal St
Boston 02114
Tel: (617) 367-8890

Michigan
Alliance for the Mentally Ill
24133 Northwest Hwy, #103
Southfield 48075
Tel: (313) 355-0010

New Jersey
Alliance for the Mentally Ill
400 Route 1, #10
Monmouth Junction 08852
Tel: (201) 329-2888

New York
Alliance for the Mentally Ill
260 Washington Ave
Albany 12210
Tel: (518) 462-2000

North Carolina
Alliance for the Mentally Ill
4900 Water Edge Dr, Suite 170
Raleigh 27606
Tel: (919) 859-2201
or 1-800-451-9682 (in NC only)

Ohio
Alliance for the Mentally Ill
55 S. Third St, #102
Columbus 43215
Tel: (614) 464-2646

Oregon
Alliance for the Mentally Ill
3000 Market St, #266
Salem 97301
Tel: (503) 370-7774

Pennsylvania
Alliance for the Mentally Ill
2149 N. Second St
Harrisburg 17110
Tel: (717) 238-1514

South Carolina
Alliance for the Mentally Ill
2016 Assembly St
Columbia
Tel: (803) 779-7849

Tennessee
Alliance for the Mentally Ill
1900 N. Winston Rd, #502
Knoxville 37919
Tel: (615) 691-3707

Texas
Alliance for the Mentally Ill
400 W. 15th St, Suite 1068
Austin 78701
Tel: (512) 474-2225

Utah
Alliance for the Mentally Ill
P.O. 26561
Salt Lake City 84126
Tel: (801) 583-2500 x2023

Vermont
Alliance for the Mentally Ill
P.O. Box 1511
Burlington 05402
Tel: 1-800-872-6488
(in Vermont only)

Virginia
Alliance for the Mentally Ill
P.O. Box 903
Richmond 23215
Tel: (804) 225-8264

The National Alliance for the
  Mentally Ill
2101 Wilson Blvd, Suite 302
Arlington 22201
Tel: (703) 524-7600

West Virginia
Alliance for the Mentally Ill
25 Clinton Hills
Tridelphia 26059
Tel: (304) 343-8850

Wisconsin
Alliance for the Mentally Ill
1245 E. Washington Ave, #212
Madison 53703
Tel: (608) 257-5888

Neuroleptics

Chlorpromazine: This is sold under a variety of trade names but is best known as Thorazine in the United States and as Largactil in other countries. It is taken in daily doses as high as 2,000 mg and as low as 25 mg. The usual daily dose is 300–1,000 mg. It commonly causes drowsiness early in treatment, though this tends to disappear after a while; drowsiness is reduced by taking all the medication in one dose at bedtime. It may also cause blurring of vision and dryness of the mouth. Some people have constipation. Parkinsonism also occurs. In many people chlorpromazine produces a sensitivity to sunlight, and people taking this drug should either stay out of the sun or else use protective clothing or barrier cream. Chlorpromazine may cause weight gain and, as with other neuroleptics, may interfere with the menstrual cycle in women, cause breast swelling, and even lactation.

Chlorprothixene (Tarasan): Rarely used, it is given in the same dosage range as chlorpromazine and thioridazine and tends to be sedative.

Flupenthixol (Fluanxol): This is a depot-injection drug used in doses of up to 200 mg. Single injections may last four weeks. Side-effects are similar to those of Modecate. It is also available in tablet form. Fluanxol has antidepressant properties, especially at low doses.

Fluphenazine: Similar to trifluoperazine in side-effects, it is used in doses up to 60 mg a day. Its original name was Moditen in Canada, Prolixin in the United States. Other brands now exist.

Fluphenazine decanoate (Modecate; Prolixin decanoate): This is a long-acting drug given by intramuscular injection. Usual maximum dosage for this drug is about 150 mg by injection every week though some people are maintained on as little as 12.5 mg every four weeks and occasionally very high weekly doses may be justified. It may cause quite marked parkinsonism and muscular restlessness. These side-effects peak two to four days following the injection. Long-acting or depot drugs such as this one make adherence to a drug schedule easier for most people.

Fluphenazine enanthate (Moditen; Prolixin enanthate): This is the original depot drug. Dosage is similar to the decanoate form but side-effects are more pronounced and it usually needs to be given more frequently. As a consequence it is now rarely used.

Fluspirilene (Imap): This drug comes as a depot injection which lasts for one or two weeks. It usually has very few side-effects. Doses up to 40 mg weekly have been used. Because it needs to be given frequently, patients may develop lumps at the injection site.

Haloperidol (Haldol): Different chemically from the drugs mentioned above, this is a potent medication which is used in dosages of up to 80 mg a day. It tends to have very similar side-effects to those of trifluoperazine. It is one of the safest drugs as far as the cardiovascular system is concerned and is often the one used for the elderly (in very small doses).

Haloperidol decanoate (Haldol LA): This is a depot-injection drug, a long-acting version of the above. Usual doses are up to 300 mg and injections may last 4 weeks. Side-effects are similar to those experienced with the oral form, although they are unexpectedly, less frequent.

Loxapine (Loxapac; Loxitane): This drug is used in dosages as high as 300 mg a day. It has generally mild side-effects which are similar to but less severe than those of trifluoperazine on the one hand and of thioridazine on the other. It has marked calming effects.

Mesoridazine (Serentil): This is a rarely used drug which tends to have more sedative and fewer parkinsonian side-effects. Average daily dose is 100 mg.

Methotrimeprazine (Nozinan): This is a rather ineffective drug useful as a sedative and used for people who develop intolerable side-effects to the stronger antipsychotics. It has a strong tendency to lower blood pressure and cause lightheadedness.

Molindone (Moban): This is said to be the only antipsychotic that does not cause weight gain. Average daily dose is 150 mg.

Pericyazine (Neuleptil): This drug has relatively few side-effects and the additional benefit of controlling obsessive thoughts. Average daily dose is 100 mg.

Perphenazine: Used in doses of up to 96 mg a day, this drug has side-effects similar to those of trifluoperazine. Its original brand name was Trilafon. Other brands are now available.

Pimozide (Orap): This drug appears to have mild side-effects and, some people claim, a reduced risk of tardive dyskinesia. It is normally used for relatively mild chronic illness. It is used in dosages of up to 20 mg a day. In higher doses it may cause heart irregularity.

Pipotiazine (Piportil): This is a depot-injection drug which can be given every four weeks. Side-effects are similar to those of Modecate. Dosage is up to 300 mg per injection.

Thioridazine: Although less expensive generic copies are now available, this drug was originally sold as Mellaril. It is used in doses similar to those of chlorpromazine but produces fewer parkinsonian side-effects than chlorpromazine. In men Mellaril sometimes causes temporary problems with erection and ejaculation. Orgasmic difficulties may also occur in women. Initially drowsiness is fairly common, as are lightheadedness, difficulty in focusing, and dry mouth. Parkinsonism is usually mild. In excessive doses it can cause heart irregularity.

Thiothixene (Navane): This drug is similar to trifluoperazine though with less severe side-effects in most people and is used in dosages of up to 80 mg a day.

Trifluoperazine: Although less expensive copies are now available, this drug was originally sold as Stelazine. It is used in dosages of up to 80 mg a day. It does not tend to cause drowsiness but does readily cause parkinsonism, restlessness, and muscular spasms. These must be counteracted by antiparkinsonian drugs.

Explanatory footnote: Parkinsonism is a common side-effect of neuroleptics, so-called because it mimics Parkinson's disease; symptoms include stiffness, tremor, restlessness, loss of arm swing, shuffling gait, blank expression.

Suggested reading

Bernheim, Kayla, and others. *The Caring Family.* New York: Random House 1982.

Dearth, Nona, and others. *Families Helping Families: Living with Schizophrenia.* New York: Norton 1986

Green, Hannah. *I Never Promised You a Rose Garden.* New York: Holt, Rinehart and Winston 1964

Tallard Johnson, Julie. *Hidden Victims: An Eight-Stage Healing Process for Families and Friends of the Mentally Ill.* Toronto: Doubleday 1988

Torrey, E. Fuller. *Surviving Schizophrenia: A Family Manual.* New York: Harper and Rowe 1983

Walsh, Maryellen. *Schizophrenia: Straight Talk for Families and Friends.* New York: William Morrow 1985

Booklets for the public

Hatfield, A. *Coping with Mental Illness in the Family: A Family Guide.* Maryland Department of Health and Mental Hygiene, 1984. This pamphlet can be purchased from the National Alliance for the Mentally Ill, 1901 North Fort Myer Drive, Suite 500, Arlington, VA 22209, USA.

Kerr, A., and others. *Schizophrenia: A Guide for Patients and Families,*

1988. This pamphlet can be purchased from the Social Work Department, Clarke Institute of Psychiatry, 250 College St., Toronto, Canada M5T 1R8; (416) 979-2221, Ext. 2576.

National Institute of Mental Health. *Schizophrenia, Questions and Answers*. U.S. Department of Health and Human Services, 1986. This pamphlet may be obtained free of charge from the National Institute of Mental Health, 5600 Fishers Lane, Rockville, MD 20858, USA.

Index